Encyclopedia of Oral and Maxillofacial Surgery

Volume III

Encyclopedia of Oral and Maxillofacial Surgery Volume III

Edited by **Dave Clark**

New Jersey

Published by Foster Academics,
61 Van Reypen Street,
Jersey City, NJ 07306, USA
www.fosteracademics.com

Encyclopedia of Oral and Maxillofacial Surgery
Volume III
Edited by Dave Clark

International Standard Book Number: 978-1-63242-003-9 (Hardback)

Printed in the United States of America.

Contents

Preface

This book has been an outcome of determined endeavour from a group of educationists in the field. The primary objective was to involve a broad spectrum of professionals from diverse cultural background involved in the field for developing new researches. The book not only targets students but also scholars pursuing higher research for further enhancement of the theoretical and practical applications of the subject.

The discipline of oral and maxillofacial surgery includes a broad range of diseases, conditions, injuries and deformities of the head, neck, face and jaws along with the hard and soft tissues of the oral cavity. It is an internationally acknowledged surgical attribute rapidly growing with new developments in technology. New handbooks are required to keep practitioners updated of the developments made world-wide. This book aims to present progressive researches on complex issues analyzed under the following sections: Advanced Oral and Maxillofacial Rehabilitation and Implantology, Orthognathic Surgery of Maxillofacial Deformities, and Temporomandibular Joint Disorders and Facial Pain.

It was an honour to edit such a profound book and also a challenging task to compile and examine all the relevant data for accuracy and originality. I wish to acknowledge the efforts of the contributors for submitting such brilliant and diverse chapters in the field and for endlessly working for the completion of the book. Last, but not the least; I thank my family for being a constant source of support in all my research endeavours.

Editor

Advanced Oral and Maxillofacial Rehabilitation and Implantology

Outfracture Osteotomy Sinus Graft: A Modified Technique Convenient for Maxillary Sinus Lifting

Jeong Keun Lee and Yong Seok Cho

Additional information is available at the end of the chapter

1. Introduction

Edentulous alveolar ridges always demonstrate atrophy when left alone without dental treatment, making rehabilitaion of masticatory function in this atrophic ridge in need of auxilliary augmentation procedures. This is always challenging in posterior maxillary edentulous area because local anatomical condition of this region is easily hampered as masticatory force in the posterior dentition and maxillary sinus is three times greater and the antrum is always subject to pneumatization; thus, facilitating the alveolar bone resorption of the maxillary sinus floor. The best way for a functional rehabilitation of the edentulous alveolar ridge is a dental implant; augmentation sinus surgery can circumvent the anatomical problems (i.e. lack of bone) associated with implant fixture installation.

Tatum introduced a surgical technique to approach the maxillary sinus [1] in 1976, when he first suggested the trapdoor approach; a new method of opening a bony window inward using a top hinge in the lateral maxillary sinus wall. Most maxillary sinuses can be accessed with this inward osteotomy technique with the exception of anatomical variations such as the presence of sinus septum in the operation field or a thick lateral maxillary sinus wall. We however, instead of inward opening, choose to move the osteotomized bony window completely out of the original site to access the Schneiderian membrane of the maxillary sinus (Fig 1). The outfractured bony segment is saved in the normal saline which will be repositioned to the original site after the completion of sinus grafting. The authors experienced excellent treatment results with this modified "outfracture osteotomy sinus grafting (OOSG)" technique which is presented herein.

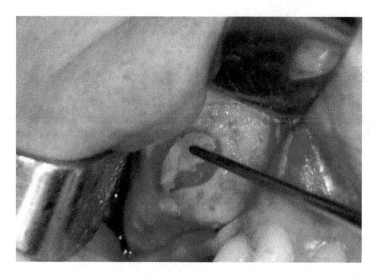

Figure 1. Outfracture osteotomy sinus grafting. The entrance to the lateral sinus wall is prepared by complete outward removal of the bony window which was carefully osteotomized by a rotary device.

2. Concept of the Outfracture Osteotomy Sinus Grafting (OOSG) technique

2.1. Conventional method

In contrast to the structural basal bone, alveolar bone is a labile bone implying it has a functional role of it which gradually degenerates following the loss of the teeth [2]. The floor of the maxillary sinus, forming the roof of the maxillary posterior alveolar bone, is always expanding downward through pneumatization especially when the alveolar bone becomes edentulous [3]. For the above two reasons, the maxillary alveolar bone is prone to atrophy when adequate tooth support is lost making problems for dentists to rehabilitate this region.

The first to introduce sinus surgery for prosthodontic preparation was Dr. Tatum. However, in 1980 Boyne and James [4] first published the detailed surgical technique and its results was for preprosthetic surgery prior to conventional prosthodontic treatment. It involved osteotomy of the lateral maxillary wall and inward fracture of the bony window with a top hinge (Fig 2). The Schneiderian membrane is elevated with this inward movement of the bony segment. It was in 1996 a consensus conference was held on sinus grafting; it was agreed that sinus grafting is an efficacious procedure and an adjunctive procedure for implant-supported restorations in the posterior maxilla [5]. Most cases are treatable with this conventional technique with the exception of some conditions.

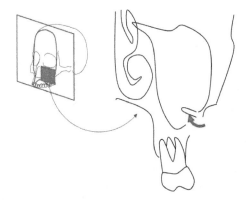

Figure 2. Concept of the original sinus approach method. It involves osteotomy of the lateral maxillary wall and inward fracture of the bony window with a top hinge.

2.2. New concept

When the lateral maxillary wall is thick enough to resist the inward force of the bony segment, sinus surgery is difficult with the conventional technique. The Schneiderian membrane may tear with excessive uncontrolled force applied to counteract this resistance. In case of sinus septae in the operative field, they may stand in way of infracture of the bony segment. The authors modified the technique to completely remove the osteotomized bony segment of the lateral wall instead of infracture and inward hinge movement. The outfractured bony segment is placed in normal saline during sinus grafting and is replaced to its original position when grafting is complete (Fig 3).

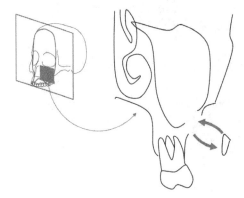

Figure 3. Concept of the outfracture osteotomy sinus grafting method. Bony window is completely removed from the lateral maxillary wall and the outfractured bony segment is placed in the normal saline during sinus grafting and is replaced to its original position before soft tissue closure.

3. Advantages and Indications of the OOSG Technique

Outfracture osteotomy sinus grafting technique is advantageous in the below situations:

1.   In cases with both height and width problems

2.   Sinus septum resisting infracture of the bony window

3.   Thick lateral sinus wall accompanying intrabony bleeding

3.1. Solution to width, as well as height problems

Essentially sinus grafting is a solution to alveolar height problems in installation of dental implant fixtures in the posterior maxillary edentulous alveolar ridges. One of the most influencing factors on the survival of the installed implant fixtures is known to be the height of the remaining alveolar bone [6]. Usually alveolar bone goes atrophic not only vertically but also transversely causing width problems in addition to height problems. In complicated cases of both height and width problems, outfracture osteotomy sinus grafting technique provides a good solution to both problems [7]. The width problem is resolved by transverse augmentation with cortical bone blocks. Outfracturing of the bony segment will secure an access to the lateral maxillary wall after elevation of the Schneiderian membrane, which will provide room for fixation screws for augmentation using cortical bone blocks (Fig 4).

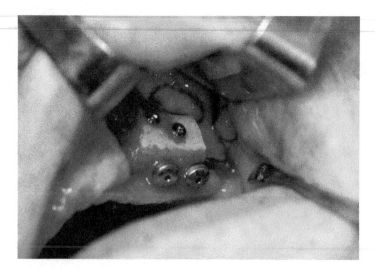

Figure 4. Outfracture osteotomy sinus grafting can be a solution to cases of both height and width problems. Complete outfracturing of the bony segment helps provide room for both sinus floor elevation and screw fixation of the cortical bone block. This patient underwent sinus grafting with OOSG technique simultaneously with a block bone graft from the mandibular ramus. Outfractured bone segment was put back to its original position before soft tissue closure.

3.2. Anatomical considerations

All cases of conventional sinus surgery are also indicated for the outfracture osteotomy sinus graft especially those with anatomic variations such as maxillary septae or a thick lateral
maxillary wall. Presurgical evaluation of the computerized tomography (CT) is useful for
the information essential to sinus surgery. Intraosseous arterial structures can be visualized
in the CT crosscut in up to 64.5 % of all maxillary sinuses [8]. Sinus septae and thick lateral
walls of the maxillary sinus is also easily visualized with CT scans, which is a good indication for outfracture osteotomy sinus grafting.

4. Surgical technique

In preparation for the simultaneous installation of the fixtures, the lateral maxillary wall is
usually accessed via crestal incision with adequate vertical extension over the buccal surface
(Fig 5). Periosteal elevation is followed by a gentle osteotomy, with the borders of the maxillary sinus imagined in mind. Osteotomy line is outlined 2mm away from the imaginary anterior and lower borders. The osteotomy line is extended with the image in mind that
antero-posteral and vertical dimension of the window is designed to be 10 mm and 5 mm,
respectively (Fig 6). Instead of usual osteotomy, the author intends a thin osteotomy line
minimizing the lost bone to help reposition the bony segment to the original position after
graft material is placed in. The usual rotary instrument is a No. 2 round carbide bur which is
adequate for minimizing bone loss (Fig 7).

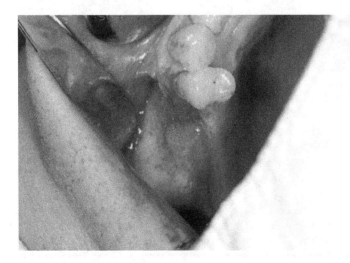

Figure 5. Lateral maxillary wall is exposed via elevation of the flap after vertical extension of the buccal side of the
aimed site which is usually accessed by crestal approach for simultaneous installation of the fixtures.

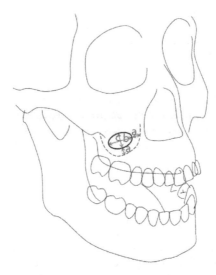

Figure 6. Osteotomy design. Imaginary border of the maxillary sinus (dashed line) is outlined based on the panoramic radiograph. Osteotomy line is designed 2mm away from the imaginary anterior and lower borders (a). The osteotomy line is extended with the image in mind that antero-posteral and vertical dimension of the window is designed to be 10 mm and 5 mm, respectively (b and c).

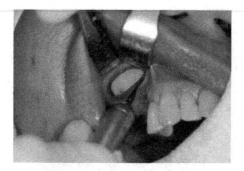

Figure 7. Exposure of the lateral maxillary wall is followed by a gentle osteotomy with rotary instrument using No. 2 round carbide bur which is adequate for minimizing bone loss. A thin osteotomy line is preferred for minimizing the lost bone to help reposition of the bony segment to the original position.

A bluish grey color beneath the osteotomy line indicates the exposure of the Schnederian membrane which must be extended along the whole osteotomy line. Usually Schneiderian membrane is identified along the osteotomy line as a bluish grey line, a landmark to stop further bone reduction not to invade the membrane surface (Fig 8). This is difficult in case of thick lateral sinus wall (to identify the bluish grey color) but instead of inward force, light outward force induces slice fragmentation of the thick lateral wall partially, just like onion skin peeling out without exposure of the Schneiderian membrane as a whole. In view of underlying remaining bone after slice outfracture, remaining bone is still thick to be removed further repeatedly until Schneiderian membrane can be seen definitely. For detailed information, please see section 5.2. and Fig 14.

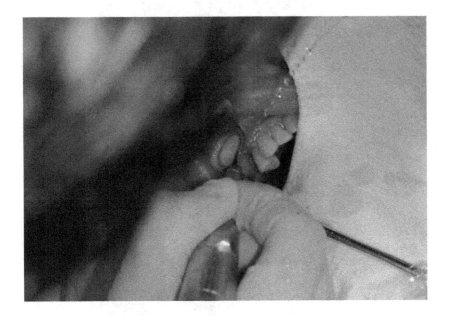

Figure 8. Osteotomy is continued until a bluish grey line is visible not to invade the Schneiderian membrane.

Outward leverage action beneath the formed bony window causes it to separate. The bony segment of the window is preserved in normal saline solution and the Schnederian membrane is undermined to separate it from the sinus floor (Fig 9). The most vulnerable stage for membrane tears is in this stage. The best way to prevent membrane perforation is to keep the tip of the sinus elevator in intimate contact with the bony floor of the maxillary sinus. The room created is filled with adequate bulk of the graft material and the bony fragment which was kept in normal saline solution is secured without any plate or screws (Fig 10). The flap is closed as usual with 4-0 Vicryl and pressure dressing for minimizing postoperative swelling.

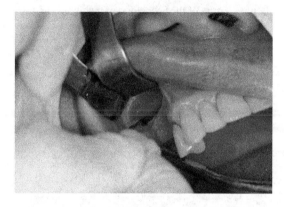

Figure 9. The Schneiderian membrane is undermined to be separated it from the sinus floor with curved sinus eleva-tors. The elevator must be kept in contact with the bony sinus floor to prevent perforation of the Schneiderian membrane.

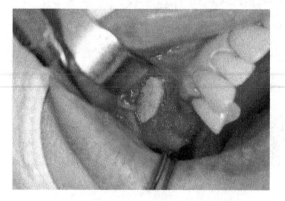

Figure 10. After the graft material is filled over the sinus floor, the bony window fragment is put back to its original position without any plate or screws followed by flap approximation with 4-0 vicryl sutures.

5. Considerations

5.1. Septum crossing the maxillary sinus

The first article on the prevalence of the septae in the maxillary sinus was in 1910 by Underwood reporting 33.0 % in 45 cadavers [9] which was an anatomical study. Varying degrees of the incidence of sinus septae, namely Underwood septae, were reported ranging from 9 % to 33.2 % [10,11,12,13,14] in clinical studies using CT scanning. Anatomical studies using cadavers demonstrated 31.7 % to 40 % of incidences [15,16,17]. Septal direction is usually buccopalatal, obstructing the inward path of the bony window in approaching the maxillary sinus (Fig 11) [14,17]. Outfracture of the bony segment can evade this problem and adequate approach becomes possible. Either two separate windows (Fig 12) or one large opening (Fig 13) can be made on the lateral wall without concern of tearing the underlying Schneiderian membrane, for there is outward leverage force instead of inward hinge movement.

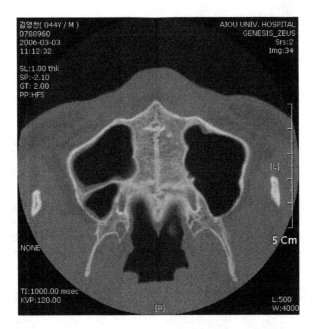

Figure 11. Typical septal structure crossing the maxillary sinus in the buccopalatal direction. It will stand in the way of sinus entry with the conventional method of inward fracturing of the bony window.

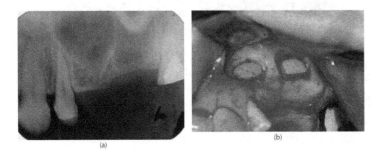

Figure 12. Sinus septum seen on a standard periapical radiograph (a), and two separate windows sinus approach (b). Separate windows can be utilized with respective outfracturing.

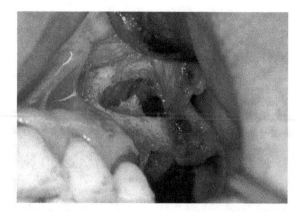

Figure 13. One large window can be utilized because of the outward, not inward vector of the segment fracturing. Septal anatomy can be identified without concerns about membrane tearing with the outfracture technique.

5.2. Thick lateral wall of the maxillary sinus

Thick lateral maxillary wall which resists inward movement is easily removed outward with only a gentle pressure. In extreme cases, the wall is fragmented out a couple of times just like onion skin peeled out one by one (Fig14 a through d). Outfracture of the thick bony segment is repeated until complete exposure of the Schneiderian membrane without concern of tearing.

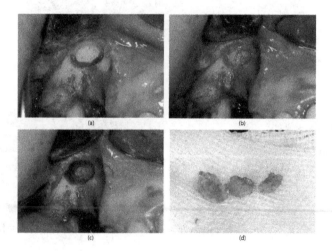

Figure 14. Repeated outfracture of the bony segments in thick lateral maxillary wall. Initial outfracture osteotomy (a) didn't succeed in revealing Schneiderian membrane (b), but continued osteotomy (c) lead to exposure of the Schneiderian membrane and left three pieces of osteotomized segments (d).

5.3. Bone bleeding during sinus approach

Head and neck structures have a high vascularity enhancing the healing capacity of this region. Extended from the external carotid artery, the internal maxillary artery feeds the maxillary sinus with its branches, infraorbital artery (IOA) and posterior superior alveolar artery (PSAA) anastomosing on the lateral maxillary wall. In a study using 100 CT scans, 94 out of 200 (47 %) examined sinuses demonstrated well-defined bony canals in the areas of sinus surgery to be done, whereas intra-osseous anastomoses of the IOA and PSAA was found by dissection in a total of 30 cadaveric maxillary sinuses [18]. Another study revealed that 52.9 % of the intraosseous branches of PSAA can be visualized on the CT scans and its average distance from the alveolar crest was demonstrated to be 16 ± 3.5 mm [19]. Typical coronal crosscut image of the CT shows the passage of the arterial structure on the lateral maxillary sinus wall as a notching inside of it (Fig 15). Adequate design of the surgical planning based on this radiographic anatomy will help prevent bleeding with outfracture osteotomy sinus graft technique because of its technical convenience.

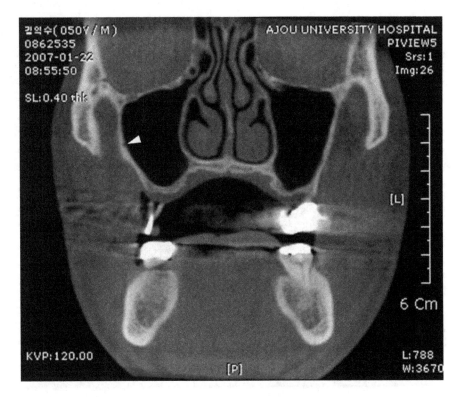

Figure 15. Crosscut image showing the notch inner cortical side of the lateral maxillary sinus wall revealing the arterial structure passing over the Schneiderian membrane (white arrowhead).

There was no vessel visible or no vessel present in most cases (120 sinuses, i.e. 89.5 %) in the cadaveric and radiographic study of 134 maxillary sinuses [20]. The other 14 cases demonstrated its appearance in two thirds of the lateral wall of the maxillary sinuses, 12 of which (85.7 %) showing vessels in the middle third. Another study showed bony canal in 114 (55 %) out of 208 CT scans in surgical planning of the maxillary sinus [21]. Because the anastomosis of the IOA and PSAA is usually in the surgical field as in these studies, surgeons approaching lateral maxillary wall encounter these vessels occasionally. During the conventional sinus approach intrabony bleeding is more difficult to deal with in the thick lateral sinus wall, for inward mobilization of the bony segment; this will be possible only after the complete reduction of the thick lateral wall. By contrast, outfracturing immediately reveals any bleeding in the surgical field. Sometimes, large arterial feature running across the surgical field can be visible after outfracturing of the bony window (Fig 16). Even in the case of thick lateral wall it may cause slice fragmentation just like an onion skin, which will not hide the bleeding in the surgical field. Surgical approach can be done with adequate bleeding control in the course of the sinus window opening.

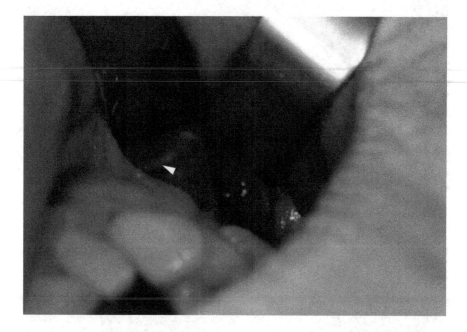

Figure 16. Large artery running across the surgical field is visible after complete removal of the bony window segment outward (white arrowhead).

5.4. Most natural covering membrane

Covering membrane is used to block access window after completion of the sinus graft procedure. In a clinical study comparing the effect of barrier membrane in the bilateral sinus floor elevation, Tarnow concluded that the barrier membrane tends to increase vital bone formation and recommended membrane placement in all sinus elevation procedures [22]. Although many kinds of barrier membranes are commercially available, outfractured bony segment functions as a covering membrane instead of artificial membrane [7,23]. It can participate in the bone remodeling procedure, for it is of self origin functioning as a natural covering membrane. It's rather a free bone graft and most of the repositioned bony segment is to take part in remodeling procedure absorbed in healing process with consolidation of graft material.

5.5. Grafting materials

Success of the bone graft depends more upon the condition of the recipient site than the kinds of the graft materials. There is little difference of success rate among various kinds of graft materials with the result of the materials used is all acceptable [5]. There are a lot of studies demonstrating many kinds of grafting materials in sinus augmentation either in animal experiment [2425] or human studies using peripheral blood [26], absorbable gelatin sponge [27], and autologous fibrin-rich block with concentrated growth factors28. Antral ossification was also reported even after Schneiderian membrane elevation without graft material in experimental studies in rabbits [24, 25]. New bone formation was also confirmed clinically, radiographically, and histologically in a human study with elevation of the Schneiderian membrane without graft material [29]. We are now grafting a material derived from autogenous teeth, the effect of which is confirmed in in-vivo study using miniature pigs [30] and by the histologic result of a human study [31].

Despite of the diverse range of treatment results of the graft materials, the overall effect of the various materials used in the sinus graft seems to be acceptable [5]. It means maxillary sinus is anatomically acceptable for graft procedure irrespective of the materials used. Maxillary sinus is a confined cavity with excellent cortical housing adequate for immobilization of the graft material, a prerequisite for an optimal healing that can induce new bone formation.

6. Fixture survival rate with outfracture osteotomy sinus graft technique

The survival of the installed implant fixture is most dependant on the initial stability of the fixture [32] and the quality of bone that takes the fixtures and not on the graft materials [33]. The conventional sinus graft technique has no advantage over the outfracture osteotomy technique, for bone segment which is trapped in is not stable to take the installed fixture.

The author has been performing sinus graft at Ajou University Hospital Dentofacial Center in Suwon, Korea when the posterior maxillary alveolar ridge is inadequate for fixture installation. All patients needing augmentation sinus surgery by lateral approach technique underwent outfracture osteotomy sinus grafting. As an independent procedure, our department has recorded 97.2 % (174 out of 179 fixtures involved in sinus graft) 5-year implant survival rate in 2009 [34]. Our overall total implant survival rate in our department was 97.9 % (751 out of 767 fixtures) with fixtures 3.75 mm in their diameters after 4.5 years [35].

As a continuing study following the previous one, a retrospective study was done on the cumulative survival rate of the fixtures. One hundred and fifty- six patients with loss of teeth and atrophy of posterior maxilla underwent augmentation sinus surgery with outfracture osteotomy sinus grafting. One hundred and fourty two out of 156 patients received simultaneous or delayed fixture installation according to our diagnostic criteria. Fixture installations were not done for the 14 patients whose implant treatments were done at respective local dental clinics. Three hundred and fourty two fixtures were installed in 142 patients and 320 fixtures were selected which fulfilled the inclusion criteria of follow-up period over 4 months. The time for follow-up ranged from a minimum of 4.2 months to a maximum of 88.2 months (average 26.8 months). The total number that underwent sinus graft surgery with outfracture osteotomy sinus graft technique was 171 (113 unilateral and 29 bilateral cases in 142 patients). Fourteen fixtures were recorded as failures, making the total cumulative survival rate 95.6 % (306 out of 320 fixtures) (Table 1). Although the cumulative survival rate was slightly less compared to the previous study [34], 171 sinuses exhibited good results without a case of major complications such as graft failure.

Age Tooth No.	Under 10	11-20	21-30	31-40	41-50	51-60	61-70	Over 70	Total
#17	0	0	0	5	20	14(1)	7	1	47(1)
#16	0	0	2	6	27(2)	17(2)	9	2	63(4)
#15	0	0	1	2	11	6	3	1	24
#14	0	0	1	1	3	4	2	0	11
#13	0	0	0	0	1(1)	1	0	0	2(1)
#23	0	0	0	0	1	1	0	0	2
#24	0	0	2	2(1)	8(1)	9	3	0	24(2)
#25	0	1	1	2	12	11	3	0	30
#26	0	0	4	11(2)	24(3)	30	7	2	78(5)
#27	0	0	2	4	13	14(1)	4	2	39(1)
Total	0	2	12	31	126	106	36	8	321

Failure cases were designated in the parentheses in relevant column.

Table 1. Total implant fixtures installed in the atrophic maxillary alveolar bone with OOSG technique.

7. Conclusion

Sinus augmentation surgery is an established procedure effective for implant-supported restorations in the posterior maxilla. Although the lateral approach to the maxillary sinus can
be done with conventional inward trapdoor method using upper hinge, the authors recommend the new method of outfracture osteotomy and repositioning of the bony window. So
called outfracture osteotomy sinus graft is technically easy and convenient for coping with
intraoperative complications such as marrow bleeding. It is a versatile method enabling the
lateral approach of the maxillary sinus even in anatomical difficulties such as the presence
of antral septae.

Author details

Jeong Keun Lee[1] and Yong Seok Cho[2]

1 Department of Dentistry Oral and Maxillofacial Surgery, Ajou University School of
Medicine, Suwon, Korea

2 Apseon Dental Hospital, Seoul, Korea

References

[1] Tatum H Jr. Maxillary and sinus implant reconstructions. Dental Clinics of North
America 1986;30(2) 207-209

[2] Lee J.K. Bone biology for implant dentistry in atrophic alveolar ridge- theory and
practice. In: Turkyilmaz I. (ed) Implant Dentistry: A Rapidly Evolving Practice. Rije-
ka: InTech; 2011. P413-434. Available from http://www.intechopen.com/books/
implant-dentistry-a-rapidly-evolving-practice/bone-biology-for-implant-dentistry-in-
atrophic-alveolar-ridge-theory-and-practice (accessed 15 August 2012).

[3] Sharan A, Madjar D. Maxillary Sinus Pneumatization Following Extractions: A Radiographic Study. International Journal of Oral and Maxillofacial Implants 2008;23(1)
48-56

[4] Boyne PJ, James R. Grafting of the maxillary sinus floor with autogenous marrow
and bone. Journal of Oral Surgery 1980;38(8) 613-616

[5] Jensen OT, Shulman LB, Block MS, Iacono VJ. Report of the sinus consensus conference of 1996. International Journal of Oral and Maxillofacial Implants 1998;13(Suppl)
11-45

[6] Froum SJ, Tarnow DP, Wallace SS et al.: Sinus floor elevation using anorganic bovine
bone matrix (OsteoGraf/N) with and without autogenous bone: a clinical, histologic,

radiographic, and histomorphometric analysis--Part 2 of an ongoing prospective study. International Journal of Periodontics and Restorative Dentistry 1998;18(6): 528-543

[7] Lee JK. Outfracture osteotomy on lateral maxillary wall as a modified sinus graft technique. Journal of Oral and Maxillofacial Surgery 2010;68(7) 1639-1641

[8] Güncü GN, Yildirim YD, Wang HL, Tözüm TF. Location of posterior alveolar artery and evaluation of maxillary sinus anatomy with computerized tomography: a clinical study. Clinical Oral Implants Research 2011;22(10) 1164-1167

[9] Underwood AS. An inquiry into the anatomy and pathology of the maxillary sinus. Journal of Anatomy and Physiology 1910;44(4) 354-369

[10] Lee DH, Lee SH, Hwang JH, Lee JK. Clinical study on the Korean posterior maxillae related to dental implant treatment. Journal of Korean Association of Maxillofacial Plastic and Reconstructive Surgeons 2010;32(1) 27-31

[11] Lee WJ, Lee SJ, Kim HS. Analysis of location and prevalence of maxillary sinus septa. Journal of Periodontal Implant Science 2010;40(2) 56-60

[12] Kim MJ, Jung UW, Kim CS, Kim KD, Choi SH, Kim CK, Cho KS. Maxillary sinus septa: prevalence, height, location, and morphology. A reformatted computed tomography scan analysis. Journal of Periodontology 2006;77(5) 903-908

[13] Park YB, Jeon HS, Shim JS, Lee KW, Moon HS. Analysis of the anatomy of the maxillary sinus septum using 3-dimensional computed tomography. Journal of Oral and Maxillofacial Surgery 2011;69(4) 1070-1078

[14] Neugebauer J, Ritter L, Mischkowski RA, Dreiseidler T, Scherer P, Ketterle M, Rothamel D, Zöller JE. Evaluation of maxillary sinus anatomy by cone-beam CT prior to sinus floor evaluation. International Journal of Oral and Maxillofacial Implants 2010;25(2) 258-265

[15] Ulm CW, Solar P, Krennmaier G, Matejka M, Watzek G. Incidence and suggested surgical management of septa in sinus-lift procedures. International Journal of Oral and Maxillofacial Implants 1995;10(4) 462-465

[16] Ella B, Noble RDa, Lauverjat Y, Sédarat C, Zwetyenga N, Siberchicot F, Caix P. Septa within the sinus: effect on evaluation of the sinus floor. British Journal of Oral and Maxillofacial Surgery 2008;46(4) 464-467

[17] Rosano G, Taschieri S, Gaudy JF, Lesmes D, DelFabbro M. Maxillary sinus septa: a cadaveric study. Journal of Oral and Maxillofacial Surgery 2010;68(6) 1360-1364

[18] Rosano G, Taschieri S, Gaudy JF, Weinstein T, Del Fabbro M. Maxillary sinus vascular anatomy and its relation to sinus surgery. Clinical Oral Implants Research 2011;22(7) 711-715

[19] Elian N, Wallace S, Cho SC, Jalbout ZN, Froum S. Distribution of the maxillary artery as it relates to sinus floor augmentation. International Journal of Oral and Maxillofacial Implants 2005;20(5) 784-787

[20] Ella B, Sédarat C, Noble RDa C, Normand E, Lauverjat Y, Siberchicot F, Caix P, Zwetyenga N. Vascular connections of the lateral wall of the sinus: surgical effect in sinus augmentation. International Journal of Oral & Maxillofacial Implants 2008;23(6) 1047–1052

[21] Mardinger O, Abba M, Hirshberg A, Schwartz-Arad D. Prevalence, diameter and course of the maxillary intraosseous vascular canal with relation to sinus augmentation procedure: a radiographic study. International Journal of Oral and Maxillofacial Surgery 2007;36(8) 735-738

[22] Tarnow DP, Wallace SS, Froum SJ, Rohrer MD, Cho SC. Histologic and clinical comparison of bilateral sinus elevations with and without barrier membrane placement in 12 patients: Part 3 of an ongoing prospective study. International Journal of Periodontics and Restorative Dentistry 2000;20(2) 117-125

[23] Cho YS, Park HK, Park CJ. Bony window repositioning without using a barrier membrane in the lateral approach for maxillary sinus bone graft; clinical and radiologic results at 6 months. International Journal of Oral and Maxillofacial Implants 2012;27(1) 211-217

[24] Sohn DS, Kim WS, An KM, Song KJ, Lee JM, Mun YS. Comparative histomorphometric analysis of maxillary sinus augmentation with and without bone grafting in rabbit. Implant Dentistry 2010;19(3) 259-270

[25] Sohn DS, Moon JW, Lee WH, Kim SS, Kim CW, Kim KT, Moon YS. Comparison of New Bone Formation in the Maxillary Sinus With and Without Bone Grafts; Immunochemical Rabbit Study. International Journal of Oral and Maxillofacial Implants 2011;26(5) 1033-1042

[26] Moon JW, Sohn DS, Heo JW, Shin HI, Jung JK. New bone formation in the maxillary sinus using peripheral venous blood alone. Journal of Oral and Maxillofacial Surgery 2011;69(9) 2357-2367

[27] Sohn DS, Moon JW, Moon KN, Cho SC, Kang PS. New bone formation in the maxillary sinus using only absorbable gelatin sponge. Journal of Oral and Maxillofacial Surgery 2010;68(6) 1327-1333

[28] Sohn DS, Heo JU, Kwak DH, Kim DE, Kim JM, Moon JW, Lee JH, Park IS. Bone Regeneration in the Maxillary Sinus Using an Autologous Fibrin-Rich Block With Concentrated Growth Factors Alone. Implant Dentistry 2011;20(5) 389-395

[29] Sohn DS, Lee JS, Ahn MR, Shin HI. New bone formation in the maxillary sinus without bone grafts. Implant Dentistry 2008;17(3) 321-331

[30] Jeong HR, Hwang JH, Lee JK. Effectiveness of autogenous tooth bone used as a graft material for regeneration of bone in miniature pig. Journal of the Korean Association of Oral and Maxillofacial Surgeons 2011;37(5) 375-379

[31] Kim YK, Kim SG, Byeon JH, Lee HJ, Um IU, Lim SC, Kim SY. Development of a novel bone grafting material using atogenous teeth. Oral Surgery, Oral Medicine, Oral Pathology, Oral Radiology, and Endodontology 2010;109(4) 496-503

[32] Albrektsson T, Brånemark PI, Hansson HA, Lindström J. Osseointegrated titanium implants. Requirements for ensuring a long-lasting, direct bone-to-implant anchorage in man. Acta Orthopaedica Scandinavica 1981; 52(2) 155-170

[33] Molly L. Bone density and primary stability in implant therapy. Clinical Oral Implants Research 2006;17(Suppl 2) 124-35

[34] Song SI, Jeong HR, Kim HM, Lee JK. Clinical investigation on the feasibility of out-fracture osteotomy sinus graft technique. Journal of the Korean Association of Oral and Maxillofacial Surgeons 2009;35(5) 367-371

[35] Ko SM, Lee JK, Eckert SE, Choi YG. Retrospective Multicenter Cohort Study of the Clinical Performance of 2-stage Implants in South Korean Populations. International Journal of Oral and Maxillofacial Implants 2006;21(5) 785-788

Chapter 2

Concepts in Bone Reconstruction for Implant Rehabilitation

Hany A. Emam and Mark R. Stevens

Additional information is available at the end of the chapter

1. Introduction

The standard of care regarding tooth loss replacement is evolving towards the use of dental implants. The practice of fixed bridges and partial prosthesis can be and are iatrogenic to the existing teeth and bone. Prosthetics in the restoration of partial and complete edentulous conditions with implants has become the most important determinant. Because of this principle the emphasis has focused on optimization of the alveolus to receive a root form implant. Dental implants are a viable treatment option when there is sufficient quantity and quality of bone to achieve the desired functional and esthetic results. The reduction in bone volume has many etiologies. The most common are a result of: Periodontal disease, pneumatization of the maxillary sinus, long term ill-fitting dentures, and the general progression of osteoporosis with aging. Initially, malposition or short implants were used in areas of deficient bone volume. This often resulted in compromised prosthetic design and poor long term treatment outcomes. Today's treatment plans first consider the prosthesis options. This necessitates reconstruction and modifications of the pre-existing anatomy provide the ideal environment needed for optimal implant placement. The deformity is often a composite loss of both bone and soft tissue. The alveolar bone loss frequently occurs in a three dimensional pattern. Multiple options and techniques have been advocated for correction and reconstruction of the atrophied alveolar bones. They include the following: Guided bone regeneration (GBR), onlay bone grafting (OBG), interpositional bone grafting (IBG), distraction osteogenesis (DO), ridge- split (RS), and sinus augmentation techniques (SA). [1-3] The complexity of the defect dictates the selection of the appropriate technique. The reconstruction must also take into account the three dimensional spatial relation of one arch to the opposing arch.

2. Considerations for reconstruction

2.1. Bone density

The quality of bone in the jaws is dependent on location and position within the dental arches and alveolus respectively. The most dense bone is observed in the anterior mandible, followed by the anterior maxilla and posterior mandible. The least compact bone is typically found in the posterior maxilla. Misch classified these bone densities into a spectrum of four categories, ranging from D1 through D4. D1 bone primarily consists of a dense cortical structure. D4 on the other hand, is the softest, consisting primarily of cancellous bone with a fine trabecular pattern with minimal crestal cortical anatomy. The density of bone is an important quality in the initial stabilization of the implant and in the loading profile of the prosthesis. Literature review of clinical studies from 1981 to 2001 reveals that poor bone density may decrease implant loading survival rates. The decrease survival ranged from 16% to 40 %. The primary cause of these failures was directly attributed to the bone density, strength and a lower percentage of bone to implant contact. Bone in the posterior maxilla was found to be five to ten times weaker in comparison to bone in the anterior when compared to other bone densities. Lesser bone densities also influence stress pattern distribution. Stresses in "soft bone" demonstrate patterns which migrate further towards the apex. Bone loss is more pronounced and occurs along the implant body rather than crestally, as in denser bone. D4 bone exhibits the greatest difference in biomechanical modulus of elasticity when compared with titanium. Therefore, afterload results in higher strain conditions at the bone-implant interface accelerating bone resorption and implant failure (Fig. 1).

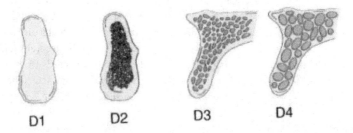

Figure 1. Types of bone densities

2.2. Bone graft materials and mechanism of bone regeneration

Various bone augmentation materials are used for alveolar reconstruction, they include: Autografts, allografts, alloplasts, and xenografts. Autogenous bone grafts can regenerate bone through all three mechanisms: *osteogenesis, osteoinduction, and osteoconduction*; This is the gold standard. Other bone substitute materials form bone from osteoinduction and or osteoconduction in varying degrees.

Osteogenesis is new bone formation. New bone forms from osteoprogenitor cells that are present in the graft. They survive the transplantation, proliferate and differentiate to osteoblasts. *This is termed phase I osteogenesis.* Autogenous bone is the only graft material with osteogenic properties. [4]

Osteoinduction involves new bone formation by stimulation and recruitment of osteoprogenitor cells derived from undifferentiated mesenchymal stem cells at the graft site, *this is called phase II osteogenesis.* The method of recruitment and differentiation occurs through a cascade of events triggered by graft- derived inducing factors called *bone morphogenic proteins* (BMP), which are members of the transforming growth factor- β superfamily. These BMPs are present in the matrix of the graft and are accessed after the mineral content of the graft has been removed by a chemical dissolution process and or osteoclastic activity. It has been shown that osteoinductive materials can induce bone formation even in ectopic sites (subcutaneous tissue). [5]

Osteoconduction is the ingrowth of the vascular tissue and mesenchymal stem cells into the scaffold structure provided by a graft material. Bone formation occurs by resorption or apposition from the existing or surrounding bone. This process is called *creeping substitution; and also classified as phase III osteogenesis.* This process must occur in the presence of vital bone or undifferentiated mesenchymal cells. Osteoconductive materials do not grow bone when placed in soft tissue. Instead, the material remains relatively unchanged or resorbs. [6]

2.3. Types of bone grafts

Autografts are grafts harvested from the individual. Autogenous bone uses all three known mechanisms of bone regeneration. They are also non immunogenic and its superiority comes from the transfer of osteocompetent cells. [7]Autogenous bone can be harvested from multiple sites within the body. The most common intra-oral sites are the symphysis, maxillary tuberosity, ramus, coronoid process, and or shavings from osteotomy preparations. The advantage of harvesting intra-orally are, ease of harvesting and the harvest site being within the same reconstruction field. The major disadvantage of intra-oral harvesting is the limited amount and quality of the harvested bone. Extra-oral bone graft harvesting is used to provide large volumes of the material and is indicated for major augmentation procedures. Iliac crests, tibia, fibula, and the cranial bone are common sites for graft harvesting. [8]

Allografts are grafts taken from the same species as the host, but is genetically dissimilar. The grafts are prepared as fresh, frozen, freeze-dried, mineralized and demineralized. There are numerous configurations of allograft bone, including powder, cortical chips, cancellous cubes, cortical struts, and others. Once the grafts are harvested, they are processed through different methods, including physical debridement, ultrasonic washing, treatment with ethylene oxide, antibiotic washing, gamma irradiation for spore elimination, and freeze drying. The goal of these steps is to remove the antigenic component and reduce the host immune response while retaining the biologic characteristics of the graft. However, the mechanical properties of the graft are often weakened (Table 1) [9]

Allogenic bone is principally osteoconductive, although, it may retain some osteoinductive capability. This quality is dependent upon how the material is processed. Urist in 1965 described the process of acid demineralization of bone before implantation by using hydro-chloric acid. The organic bone matrix contains bone morphogenic proteins (BMPs). These proteins are responsible for the de novo bone formation. BMP is not acid soluble, however the calcium and phosphate salts of the HA can be removed from the bone in the acid- reducing process. This results in demineralization of the freeze-dried bone (FDB) and an increased exposure of the BMPs with its osteopromotive effect. FDB is primary osteoconductive while demineralized freeze dried bone (DFDB) is believed to be osteoinductive. [10] Results of studies performed using DFDB are conflicting. Controversy still exists about the osteopromo-tive effects of DFDB. Some reports raise the question of the concentration variability of BMPs in commercially available grafts. Osteoinductive properties of DFDB vary from one cadaver to another. The product fabrication may also have an effect on the osteoinductivity of the allograft where the demineralization process is very technique sensitive. For example, it has been shown that the osteoinductive properties of the grafts are removed, if the calcium content is less than 2% by weight. In addition, controversy persists about the use of ethylene oxide for sterilization of the graft materials and its possible destructive affects on the BMPs. [11]Dem-ineralized cortical bone was found to have higher concentrations of BMPs than trabecular bone. Membranous cortical bone exhibits greater concentration of BMPs than endochondral cortical bone, consequently; the skull and facial bone represent a better source of inductive proteins than the remaining appendicular skeleton.

Routine studies are performed to evaluate the safety of allografts. According to the American association of tissue banks the probability of DFDB to contain HIV virus is 1 in 2.8 billion. When compared with the risk of 1 in 450,000 for blood transfusions, the risk of infection from allografts seems infinitesimal. Rigorous background checks are performed on the donor and his/her family before the donor is accepted into the program. Occasionally biopsy specimens of sites containing allograft from human patients sometimes show chronic inflammatory cells. These histologic appearances of a non-specific inflammatory condition cannot be attributed to an immune reaction with certainty.[6]

Xenografts are derived from the inorganic portion of bone of a genetically different species than the host. One of the most popular used xenografts is the bovine bone. It is a good bone bank material. The process requires complete de-proteinization at high temperature, (1100 °c). This results in total removal of the residual organics that might provoke an immune response (Table 2). [12]

A concern over the risk of disease transmission from cattle to humans through the bone graft material derived from bovine bone used for dental implants has been suggested. The recent incidents of *bovine spongiform encephalopathy* (BSE) in human have underscored this likelihood. Results from analysis conducted by the German Federal Ministry of Health and by the Pharmaceutical Research and Manufacturers Association of America showed that the risk of disease transmission was negligible and could be attributed to the stringent protocols followed in sourcing and processing of the raw bovine bone used in the commercial products. [13] One of the best known xenografts is *Bio-Oss* (Osteohealth, Shirley, NY). It has been treated by having all its organic material removed. This leaves a crystal structure that practically matches human cancellous bone in structure. In 1992, Klinge and colleagues, noted total resorption of Bio-Oss granules at 14 weeks after placement in rabbit skulls. [14] However, Skoglund and colleagues reported that granules were present even after 44 months [15].

Another popular alternative xenograft is *coralline hydroxyapatite*, which is made from ocean corals. This material was created with the intension of producing a graft material with a more consistent pore size. Coral, which is composed mainly of calcium carbonate, is processed to remove most of the organic content. Then it is subjected to high pressure and heat in the presence of an aqueous phosphate solution. When this process is completed, the calcium carbonate skeleton is totally replaced with a calcium phosphate skeleton (hydrothermal exchange). The material is concurrently sterilized in this process. [16] The generation of biomimetic microenvironments, using scaffolds containing cell recognition sequences in combination with bone cells, offers tremendous potential for skeletal tissue regeneration. *PepGen P15* (DENTSPLY Friadent CeraMed, Lakewood, CO) is the first man engineered collagen I binding domain for potential osteoblasts and is able to multiply the complete regeneration cascade (Figs. 2,3). It is a combination bone replacement graft material composed of natural anorganic bovine-derived hydroxyapatite matrix (ABM) coupled with a synthetic cell-binding peptide (P-15). [17]

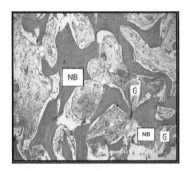

Figure 2. Microphotograph (16 weeks 5x 1.25 OP H&E) showing newly formed bone (NB) in an interconnecting trabecular pattern (bone bridging) surrounding the remaining graft particles G. (PepGen P-15).

Alloplasts are synthetic bone substitutes that posses osteoconductive potential. The ideal synthetic graft material should be biocompatible and elicit minimal fibrotic changes. The graft should support new bone growth and undergo remodeling. Other preferred attributes would include similar toughness, modulus of elasticity, and compressive strength compared to that of the host cortical or cancellous bone. Many synthetic materials are available including: Bioactive glasses, glass ionomers, aluminum oxide, calcium sulphate, calcium phosphates as α and β tricalcium phosphate (TCP), synthetic hydroxyapatite (HA), and synthetic absorbable polymers. [16] Synthetic bone substitutes offer many advantages; however, the greatest is the unlimited supply and avoidance of a secondary surgical procedure. The main disadvantage is the material's lack of the osteoinductive capabilities, experienced in autogenous grafts. Clinicians may prefer performing grafting procedures using *combination grafts*. This will combine the osteogenic potential of autogenous bone with the unlimited supply offered by

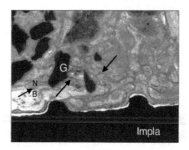

Figure 3. Microphotograph (8 weeks 5x 1.6 OP Paragon) showing the newly formed bone (NB) in an interconnecting trabecular pattern (bone bridging-arrows) surrounding the remaining graft particles G (PepGen P-15) supporting a dental implant.

bone substitutes which act as *expanders* or *fillers*. Combination grafts also minimize donor site morbidity that occurs more frequently when harvesting larger volumes of autogenous bone (Table 3).

Allografts

Material	Commercial source	composition	Bone Growth Method	Resorption time
DFDB (Demineralized)	Pacific Tissue Bank Grafton MTF DynaGraft	Collagen + Growth factors	Mainly Osteoinduction varies based upon processing method	+/- 6 months
FDB (Mineralized)	MinerOss Puross	Minerals + Collagen	Mainly Osteoconduction	1 Yr +

Table 1.

Xenografts

Material	Brand name	Structure
Deprotenized bovine bone mineral	Bio-Oss	Cancellous or cortical
Anorganic bovine HA+ cell binding peptide	PepGen P-15	Peptide + microporous HA
	Osteograft N	Micro + Macroporous
Coral (Ca carbonate)	Biocoral Interpore 200 (Coralline)	Natural coral

Table 2.

Alloplasts	
Ceramics	**Polymers**
β-tricalcium phosphate (β-TCP)	Methylmethacrylate (HTR synthetic bone)
Hydroxyapatite (HA), (Bone source, Norian)	Poly- α- hydroxy acids (PLA,PLGA)
Ca2So4 (Plaster of paris)	
Calcium phosphate cements (Ceredex, α-BSM)	
Bioactive glass (PerioGlass, BioGran)	

Table 3.

2.4. Properties of graft materials

It is important to consider the physical and chemical properties of the graft materials used in the augmentation procedures. *Physical properties* include the surface area or form of the product (block, particle), porosity (dense, macroporous, microporous), and crystallinity (crystalline, amorphous). *Chemical properties* are related to calcium –to- phosphorous ratio, element impurities (such as carbonate), and the pH of the surrounding region. These properties play a role in the rate of resorption and clinical applications of the material.[7] The larger the particle size, the longer the material will remain at the augmentation site. It was also reported that the greater the porosity, the more rapid the resorption of the graft material as this will give the chance for committed cells and blood vessels (bone modeling unit) to invade the spaces between the graft particles replacing the graft with the newly formed bone. However, dense HA may lack any micro or macro porosity within the particles with long resorption rate since the osteoclasts only attack the surface and cannot penetrate the dense material. With respect to crystallinity, the higher the crystalline structure the harder for the body to break down and absorb it.[7] The resorption of bone substitutes may be cell or solution- mediated. Cell mediated resorption requires living cells of the body to resorb the material mainly osteoclasts. A solution –mediated resorption is a chemical process; impurities like calcium carbonate permit solution – mediated resorption, which then increases the porosity of the graft. The pH in the region also affects the rate of graft resorption. As the pH decreases (due to infection) the HA components resorb by a solution – mediated resorption. Bone, dense HA, macroporous HA, microporous HA, crystalline HA, or amorphous HA may all resorb within a two-week period (Fig. 4).[7]

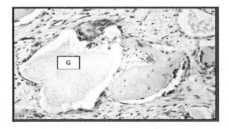

Figure 4. Showing the cell - mediated resorption of multinucleated cells (arrow) on the surface of the graft particle (G).

Close matching of the resorption rate to the bone deposition rate is important. Selection of graft material should be based on location of graft site, soft tissue environment, and its possible role in promoting and supporting future implant osseous integration. A rapidly resorbing scaffold might reestablish a void filled with connective tissue, whereas one that resorb too slowly, or not at all, would impede bone deposition and limit creeping substitution. There are, however clinical indications in which resorption is not desired, but rather, a permanent implant is preferred, such as craniofacial onlays for cosmetic augmentation.

2.5. Bone growth factors

The term growth factors comprises a group of polypeptides of approximately 6-45 KD (kilo Dalton) which are involved in cellular proliferation, differentiation and morphogenesis of tissues and organs during embryogenesis, postnatal growth, and adulthood. [18] Factors that are involved in the regeneration and induction of bone tissue have attracted attention as they possibly can facilitate skeletal reconstruction. These factors include platelet derived growth factor (PDGF), vascular endothelial growth factor (VEGF), insulin like growth factors (IGF), transforming growth factor β (TGF β), bone morphogenic proteins (BMPs), and platelet rich plasma (PRP).

Bone morphogenic proteins (BMPs), particularly BMP2, BMP4 and BMP7, appear to be the most reliable factors of all growth factors currently discussed with regard to enhancement of bone regeneration in reconstruction of the facial skeleton (Table 4). BMPs stimulate angiogenesis, migration, proliferation, and differentiation of mesenchymal stem cells into bone forming cells in the area of bone injury. Although a high washout effect of BMP during the first few hours in most of the carriers used has to be taken into account, this short-term signal appears to be sufficient for the initial induction of the cascade of endochondral bone formation to provide bone regeneration in the defects of the various models. Recombinant techniques are now used to provide large amounts of BMPs which are normally present in very small quantities within the organic matrix of bone (accounting for only approximately 0.1% of the mass of the organic matrix). [19] Bioactive Proteins, GEM 21S® is a combination of a bioactive proteins (highly purified recombinant human platelet derived growth factor, rhPDGF-BB) and a biocompatible osteoconductive matrix (beta-tricalcium phosphate, β-TCP). It is presently being used for periodontal regeneration procedures and offers a greater amount of growth factors as normally found in Platelet Rich Plasma (PRP).

The apparent strong desire of clinicians for the use of growth factors to facilitate reconstructive surgical procedures by obviating the need for procurement of autogenous grafts is contrasted by their limited availability for clinical application. This has prompted the application of autogenous growth factors by using *platelet rich plasma (PRP)* derived from the patient's own blood. This preparation has come widely into use recently, despite the fact that currently there is controversial scientific evidence about the benefit of using this preparation, especially, in reconstructive and preprosthetic bone grafting. According to the characteristics of the growth factors that are present in PRP and assigned for its biological activity, the use of PRP is supposed to increase proliferation of undifferentiated mesenchymal cells and to enhance angiogenesis, which then can support bone graft incorporation by enhancing of osteoprogenitor cells in the graft. It may as well improve soft tissue healing by increasing proliferation and matrix synthesis. [20] Recently, inorder to improve the handling characteristics of the graft materials to facilitate its use in several clinical situations, several commercial suppliers have begun to provide several matrices and delivery systems as carriers. The addition of the carrier changed the consistency of the material from a particulate consistency to a more coherent hydrogel form (flow) or clay like (putty) form with ease in handling during surgical application. The carrier must be nontoxic and biocompatible and should not impede any of the steps of the bone-forming cascade. Also, when used with growth factors they must first bind to them, permit their timed release, facilitate invasion of blood vessels and enable cellular attachment, finally promoting the deposition of new bone. Sodium hyaluronate, carboxymethylcellulose, poly-α- hydroxy acids, absorbable collagen sponges (ACS) and Lecithin are among the carrier materials used. In addition to the handling characteristics, it is assumed that the carrier material when added to a particulate graft will provide spaces between these particles (lower packing density), facilitating the capillary in-growth and the creeping substitution process leading to proper healing with optimum new bone formation in a shorter period of time.

BMPs approved for clinical use and indications
rhBMP-2 (Wyeth/Medtronic)
InductOs (CHMP approved)
Open tibia fracture, 2002
Interbony spinal fusion, 2005
INFUSE Bone Graft (FDA approved)
Interbony spinal fusion, 2002
Open tibia fracture, 2004
Oral/Maxillofacial, 2007
rhOP-1 (Stryker)
OP-1 Implant (FDA HDE & CHMP approved)
Recalcitrant long bone nonunions, 2001/2004
OP-1 Putty (FDA HDE approved)
Osteolateral (intertransverse) lumbar spinal fusion revision, 2004.
Bioactive proteins Gem 21S (Osteohealth), Periodontal defects

Table 4.

3. Treatment plan for bone augmentation

The treatment planning sequence for implant dentistry begins with the design of the final prosthesis. After the determination of the type of restoration, number and position of teeth to be restored and the patients force factors are then evaluated. The bone density in the region of the implant placement is then considered. The key implant positions and the number and ideal implant sizes are then selected. Finally the available bone volume is evaluated for implant placement according to the proposed treatment plan. Previous studies have shown that the most common cause of implant failures are stress-related failures especially after loading. Mechanical stress can have both positive and negative consequences for bone tissue and, thereby, also for maintaining osseointegration of oral implants. Dental implants function to transfer occlusal loads to the surrounding biological tissues. If occlusal loads are within the bone physiologic tolerance zone, osseointegration will be maintained. On the other hand, if occlusal loads are excessive and beyond the bone physiologic tolerance limit, bone will ultimately resorb and failure of osseointegration result. Thus, as a general rule the goal of treatment planning should be to minimize and evenly distribute the mechanical stress in the implant system and the surrounding bone. [21] The magnitude of stress depends on two variables which are: The *force magnitude* that is hard to control by the dentist and the *functional cross-sectional area* which participate in load bearing and stress dissipation. This area should be considered when executing the treatment plan, where it should be adequate to allow optimum stress distribution and prevent stress concentration around dental implants. There are three types of forces may be imposed on dental implants within the oral environment namely compression, tension and shear forces. Bone is strongest when loaded via compression, 30% weaker when loaded via tension and 65% weaker when loaded with shear forces. Considering the *direction* of applied occlusal loads during implant placement is important; implants should be aligned in the oral cavity to convert these loads into more favorable compressive loads at the bone-implant interface. Therefore, in the treatment plan, implants should be oriented to receive axial forces parallel to the long axis of the implants as much as possible to avoid the destructive effects of angled forces. [22], [23]

3.1. Rationale for bone augmentation

From the previous discussion sufficient amount of bone volume should be available to provide the optimum biomechanical foundation for implant placement. Sufficient bone volume will allow placement of wide diameter implants with sufficient length and number as needed by the treatment plan instead of using small sized, short implants that were only used because of insufficient bone volume compromising the treatment outcome. Adequate bone volume allows placement and alignment of implants with optimum axial inclination to receive occlusal forces in a more favorable axial direction. In addition to providing optimum bone volume, bone augmentation procedures offered a solution in the avoidance of injuring vital structures that were present as obstacles when considering implant therapy as a treatment option, such as close proximity to the inferior alveolar canal and the maxillary sinus. It is worth mentioning that proper selection of the implant design is of paramount importance in achieving long term success. [24] Some areas in the oral cavity require special considerations, like the poor density maxillary posterior edentulous area. Wide diameter, threaded implants with optimum length should be used to increase the bone to implant contact ratio and the surface area, allowing proper stress distribution at the bone implant interface. This can only be done in the presence of sufficient bone volume to accommodate the selected implants otherwise bone augmentation procedures are mandatory. When considering esthetics, sufficient bone volume is also necessary to achieve the desirable aesthetic outcome especially in the aesthetic (anterior) zone. The emergence profile is greatly dependant on the bone surrounding dental implants allowing optimum soft tissue drape around the abutments for ideal esthetic results. Also, the presence of sufficient bone volume allows flexibility in choosing the properly sized implant for better abutment emergence profile. [25]

4. Bone augmentation techniques

4.1. Socket preservation/ Guided bone regeneration

Physiologic bone resorption results in unpredictable loss of bone following teeth extraction. This can lead to less than ideal bone volume available for implant placement especially in prolonged cases of edentulism. Multiple types of grafting materials have been used to fill the extraction sockets immediately after extraction in order to maintain the space of the extraction site and prevent its collapse. This will allow for more organized bone healing maintaining the bone height and width necessary for implant placement. Following grafting the socket, barrier membranes are used to provide guided bone regeneration by protecting the underlying grafted site during healing from undesirable cellular population from the overlying soft tissues that might compromise the outcome (Figs. 5,6).

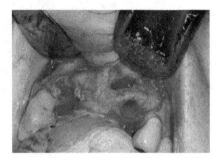

Figure 5. Socket preservation following teeth extraction.

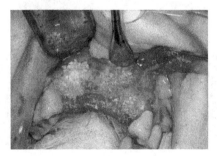

Figure 6. Grafting particulate bone

4.2. Block bone grafting technique

Block grafting approaches can be used to reconstruct significant deficiency in the vertical and horizontal dimensions of the alveolar ridge. Autogenous block grafting procedures remain the gold standard for ridge augmentation. However, donor site morbidity associated with graft harvest has turned the attention to using allogenic grafting materials. The locations for harvesting intraoral block grafts include the external oblique ridge of the posterior mandible (ramus), symphysis. With bone defects >2 cm, an extraoral donor site is warranted for harvesting larger bone volumes. The iliac crest (anterior and posterior), cranium, or tibia is often used as extraoral harvest sites. The detailed description of the harvesting techniques is beyond the scope of this chapter. Case reports have demonstrated success with FDBA and DFDBA block graft material. However, further research is warranted to evaluate the healing of these blocks histologically (Figs. 7-12).

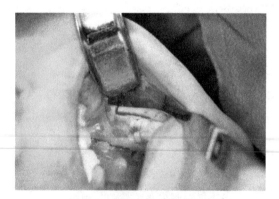

Figure 7. Ramus bone harvest

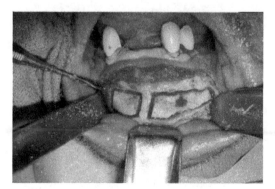

Figure 8. Symphysis bone harvest

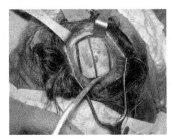

Figure 9. Calvarial bone harvest

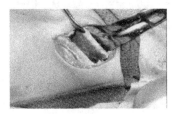

Figure 10. Anterior iliac crest bone harvest

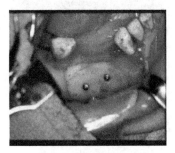

Figure 11. Mandibular bone augmentation using block. grafts. Two screws are used to prevent rotation.

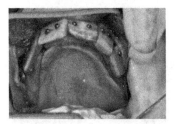

Figure 12. Maxillary ridge augmentation.

4.3. Ridge expansion (split) technique

With a narrow ridge, splitting the alveolar bone longitudinally, using chisels, osteotomes, or peizosurgical devices, can be performed to increase the horizontal ridge with, provided the facial and lingual plates are not fused and some intervening bone is present. With adequate stability of the mobile segment, sufficient interpositional grafting and soft tissue protection, comparable results to alternate techniques can be obtained. The decision to place the implants simultaneously with the split procedure or delayed placement following bone healing depend on the degree of stability of the expanded segment and the volume of remaining bone (Figs. 13-17).

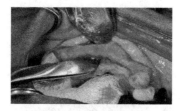

Figure 13. Narrow maxillary ridge.

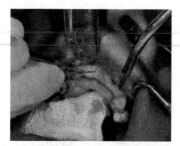

Figure 14. Osteotomy of the ridge

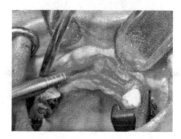

Figure 15. Ridge splitting.

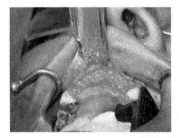

Figure 16. Interpositioning graft between the buccal and the palatal plates of bone. Collagen membrane is used to cover the expanded site

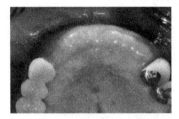

Figure 17. The augmented maxillary ridge 5 weeks postoperatively

4.4. Sinus augmentation

The most commonly used technique use to access the maxillary sinus is the lateral window technique modifying the Caldwell-Luc operation, also called the hinge osteotomy technique, originally described by Tatum then first published by Boyne and James.

A window is then created using a round bur on the lateral wall of the sinus till the bluish hue of the sinus membrane reveals itself. Using specially designed sinus elevation curettes the sinus membrane is elevated from the bony floor and is freed anteriorly, posteriorly and medially to create a tension free elevation to minimize the possibility of perforation. The trap door (window) is intruded medially forming the new sinus floor and the space created below it is then grafted to provide the platform for implant placement. The flap is then repositioned and closed. Implants are placed either simultaneously with the graft (one- stage) or after a delayed period of up to 8 months to allow for graft maturation (two- stage). The decision about the two options mainly depends on the preexisting residual amount of bone required for initial primary stability of an implant. It was found that if the bone thickness is 4 mm or less, initial implant stability would be jeopardized. In 1994, Summers published a new less invasive conservative technique for sinus floor elevation using osteotomes in an attempt to overcome the drawbacks of the lateral window approach. The technique begins with a crestal incision to expose the alveolar ridge. An osteotome of the smallest size is then tapped into place by a mallet into the bone just shy from the sinus membrane fracturing and moving the sinus floor superiorly. Osteotomes of increasing sizes are introduced sequentially to expand the alveolus and with each insertion of a larger osteotome, bone is compressed, pushed laterally and apically. Summers stated that the very nature of this technique improved the bone density of the posterior maxilla. Bone graft material is then introduced via the osteotomy followed by implant fixture insertion. The implant fixture should be slightly larger in diameter than the osteotomy site "tenting" the elevated maxillary sinus membrane. A minimally invasive antral membrane balloon elevation (MIAMBE) which is a modification of the osteotome technique has also been introduced with satisfactory results. It comprises the introduction of a balloon into the osteotomy site which is then slowly inflated to elevate the sinus membrane. This procedure showed predictable results and required a short learning curve. Recently, some authors have reported the use of a piezoelectric device in maxillary sinus surgery. Ultrasound has been increasingly used in many fields of medicine such as tumor enucleation, fragmentation of renal calculi and lithotripsy of gall bladder stones. Ultrasonic dissection has been classified as tissue-selective technique that might improve the efficiency of dissections and at the same time reduces the morbidity rate resulting from iatrogenic injuries. In addition, ultrasound energy can induce a cavitational effect in water containing tissues, which can in turn facilitate the tissue separation (Figs. 18,19).

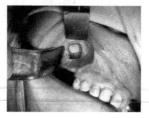

Figure 18. Showing the lateral window approach

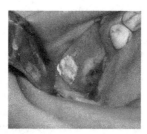

Figure 19. Sinus augmentation with immediate implant placement

4.5. Distraction osteogenesis

Distraction Osteogenesis (DO) uses the phenomenon that new bone fills in the gap defect created when two pieces of bone are slowly separated under tension. Distraction of the segment can be achieved in a vertical and /or horizontal direction on the basic principles involved in distraction which include a latency period of 7 days for initial soft callus formation, a distraction phase during which the 2 segments of bone undergo incremental gradual separation at a rate ~ 1 mm per day to stretch the formed soft callus, and a consolidation phase that allows healing of the regenerated bone between the 2 segments. The prerequisites for optimal bone augmentation of defects using DO are minimum of 6-7 mm of bone height above vital structures, such as neurovascular bundles or air passages/sinus cavities, a vertical ridge defect of > 3 -4 mm, and an edentulous span of three or more missing teeth (Figs. 20,21).

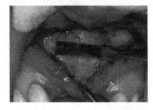

Figure 20. Alveolar distraction of the anterior maxillary region

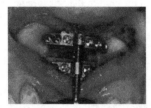

Figure 21. Note: the vertical osteotomy cuts should be divergent to avoid obstructing the path of distracting the transport segment.

4.6. Tent- Pole technique

Marx et al in 2002 advanced the approach of soft tissue matrix expansion using corticocancellous bone grafting with dental implants to treat severely resorbed mandibles that were shorter than 6 mm. Using this transcutaneous submental approach, 4 to 6 dental implants were placed to act as "tent poles" to maintain the height of the overlying mucosal soft tissue and prevent it from sagging around the iliac crest graft (Figs. 22, 23). [2]

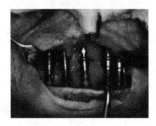

Figure 22. Implant placement in the severely atrophic mandible through a submental approach

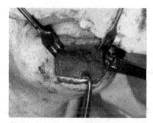

Figure 23. Corticocancellous bone graft around the implants tenting the soft tissue

4.7. Bone ring technique

Three dimensional bone augmentations with immediate dental implant placement can be done using this technique. Using trephine burs corresponding to the extraction socket diameters, bone rings can be harvested from the chin or iliac crest regions. The harvested rings can then be secured to the extraction socket using the dental implants restoring the deficient bone at the crestal portion in a 3D fashion (Figs. 24,25). [27]

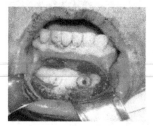

Figure 24. Three dimensional crestal bone augmentation using bone rings.

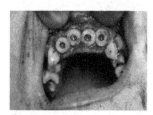

Figure 25. Immediate implant placement in the anterior maxilla

4.8. Reconstruction of segmental bony defects

Ablative loss of both bone and associated soft tissue from treatment of neoplastic or other pathologic processes represent a far different task from loss of bone from physiologic resorption, trauma or infection. The goals of reconstruction are to restore jaw continuity, provide morphology and position of the bone in relation to its opposing jaw, provide adequate height and width of bone, and provide facial contour and support for soft tissue structures.

Graft malpositioning result in occlusal problems and presents a formidable task to the restorative dentist. The site of the graft harvest depends mainly on the size of the residual defect (Figs. 26-28).

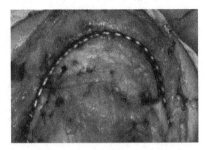

Figure 26. Reconstruction plate in place.

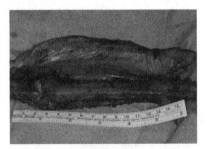

Figure 27. Free fibula graft.

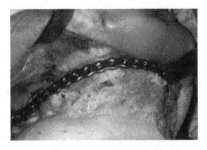

Figure 28. Reconstruction of mandibular segmental bone defect using free fibula.

4.9. Combination grafts

In large defects, the use of grafting materials from different sources can be beneficial. Some techniques aim to combine the osteogenic potential of autogenous bone with the osteocon-ductive and space maintaining properties provided by the allogenic or alloplastic sources. Allogenic materials can provide constructs that are close in morphology as the resected part providing superior esthetic outcome following the grafting procedure (Fig. 29,30).

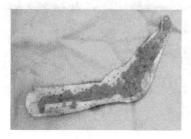

Figure 29. Hemimandibular reconstruction using a cadaveric mandible in combination with cancellous bone graft harvested from the iliac crest.

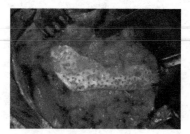

Figure 30. Graft in position.

4.10. Future augmentation approaches

Future bone augmentation approaches likely will use molecular, cellular, and genetic tissue engineering technologies. Gene therapy is a relatively new therapeutic modality based on the potential for delivery of altered genetic material to the cell. Localized gene therapy can be used to increase the concentration of desired growth or differentiation factors to enhance the regenerative response. Cellular tissue engineering strategies that include the in vitro amplifi-cation of osteoprogenitor cells grown within three dimensional constructs is currently of particular interest. The use of mesenchymal stem cell for construct seeding showed promise for bone regeneration. These approaches may lead to further refinement and improvement in alveolar bone augmentation techniques.

5. Surgical caveats for bone grafting

There are several factors that may improve the success and predictability of bone graft procedures, they include the following:

5.1. Surgical asepsis and absence of infection

Contamination of bone grafts due to endogenous bacteria, lack of aseptic surgical technique, inadequate soft tissue closure and salivary exposure may lead to infection with subsequent lowering of the pH. Solution –mediated resorption will follow with resultant graft loss. Some clinicians prefer including antibiotics locally within the graft materials to guard against bacterial contamination as no blood supply is present early in the graft. Primary soft tissue closure is also mandatory for the success of the grafting procedure. It allows healing by primary intension protecting the graft from any surrounding contamination until healing. Dehiscence with graft loss is one of the most common complications in bone grafting procedures. There-fore, careful surgical flap planning which ensures adequate blood supply to the site with minimal trauma and primary soft tissue closure without tension are required.

5.2. Space maintenance

Creation of a desired contoured space for bone formation is very important in the grafting procedure. If the graft material resorbs too rapidly compared with the time required for bone formation, the site may fill with connective tissue rather than bone. Therefore, the space must be maintained long enough without collapse for bone to fill the desired area. Titanium-reinforced barrier membranes, tent screws elevated above the bone at the desired height covered by a membrane, block grafts (covered by membrane or not) are all used to create and maintain space for bone growth.

5.3. Graft stability

For predictable bone augmentation, graft stability is a paramount. Bone remodeling and graft healing requires rigid interface for blood clot adhesion with its associated growth factors. If a graft become mobile its vascularity will be compromised followed by fibrous encapsulation and often sequestrate. If block grafts are used fixation can be achieved using titanium screws or the graft can be fixed using the inserted implants itself. If particulate graft is used, it can be covered with a barrier membrane fixed with membrane tacks to avoid dislodgement of the graft particles.

5.4. Regional acceleratory phenomenon (RAP)

The host site during bone augmentation procedures should be decorticated to establish bleeding points in the cortical bone prior to graft placement. This procedure will provide access for trabecular bone vessels, encourage revascularization, bring growth factors to the graft site and increase the availability of osteogenic cells promoting graft union and shorten the healing time.

Acknowledgements

The authors would like to extend their gratitude and acknowledgement to **Drs. Solon Kao DDS and Henry "Butch" Ferguson DMD**, for allowing the use of several clinical surgical cases. Their photographic documentation of specific bone grafts and regenerative techniques was instrumental in providing comprehensive examples of implant site reconstructions.

Author details

Hany A. Emam[1,2] and Mark R. Stevens[1]

*Address all correspondence to: hemam@georgiahealth.edu; mastevens@georgiahealth.edu

1 Oral and Maxillofacial Surgery Department, Georgia Health Sciences University, Augusta, Georgia, USA

2 Oral and Maxillofacial Surgery, Cairo University, Egypt

References

[1] Aghaloo, T. L, & Moy, P. K. Which hard tissue augmentation techniques are the most successful in furnishing bony support for implant placement? Int J Oral Maxillofac Implants (2007). Suppl:, 49-70.

[2] Jensen, J, Sindet-pedersen, S, & Oliver, A. J. Varying treatment strategies for reconstruction of maxillary atrophy with implants: results in 98 patients. J Oral Maxillofac Surg (1994). discussion 16-8., 52(3), 210-6.

[3] Isaksson, S, & Alberius, P. Maxillary alveolar ridge augmentation with onlay bone-grafts and immediate endosseous implants. J Craniomaxillofac Surg (1992). , 20(1), 2-7.

[4] Giannoudis, P. V, Dinopoulos, H, & Tsiridis, E. Bone substitutes: an update. Injury (2005). Suppl 3:S, 20-7.

[5] Browaeys, H, Bouvry, P, & De Bruyn, H. A literature review on biomaterials in sinus augmentation procedures. Clin Implant Dent Relat Res (2007). , 9(3), 166-77.

[6] Khan, S. N, & Cammisa, F. P. Jr., Sandhu HS, Diwan AD, Girardi FP, Lane JM. The biology of bone grafting. J Am Acad Orthop Surg (2005). , 13(1), 77-86.

[7] Misch, C. E, & Dietsh, F. Bone-grafting materials in implant dentistry. Implant Dent (1993). , 2(3), 158-67.

[8]   Clavero, J, & Lundgren, S. Ramus or chin grafts for maxillary sinus inlay and local onlay augmentation: comparison of donor site morbidity and complications. Clin Implant Dent Relat Res (2003). , 5(3), 154-60.

[9]   Marx, R. E. Bone and bone graft healing. Oral Maxillofac Surg Clin North Am (2007). v., 19(4), 455-66.

[10] Wikesjo, U. M, Sorensen, R. G, Kinoshita, A, & Wozney, J. M. RhBMP-2/alphaBSM induces significant vertical alveolar ridge augmentation and dental implant osseointegration. Clin Implant Dent Relat Res (2002). , 4(4), 174-82.

[11] Zhang, M, & Powers, R. M. Jr., Wolfinbarger L, Jr. Effect(s) of the demineralization process on the osteoinductivity of demineralized bone matrix. J Periodontol (1997). , 68(11), 1085-92.

[12] Kao, S. T, & Scott, D. D. A review of bone substitutes. Oral Maxillofac Surg Clin North Am (2007). vi., 19(4), 513-21.

[13] Sogal, A, & Tofe, A. J. Risk assessment of bovine spongiform encephalopathy transmission through bone graft material derived from bovine bone used for dental applications. J Periodontol (1999). , 70(9), 1053-63.

[14] Klinge, B, Alberius, P, Isaksson, S, & Jonsson, J. Osseous response to implanted natural bone mineral and synthetic hydroxylapatite ceramic in the repair of experimental skull bone defects. J Oral Maxillofac Surg (1992). , 50(3), 241-9.

[15] Skoglund, A, Hising, P, & Young, C. A clinical and histologic examination in humans of the osseous response to implanted natural bone mineral. Int J Oral Maxillofac Implants (1997). , 12(2), 194-9.

[16] Moore, W. R, Graves, S. E, & Bain, G. I. Synthetic bone graft substitutes. ANZ J Surg (2001). , 71(6), 354-61.

[17] Nguyen, H, Qian, J. J, Bhatnagar, R. S, & Li, S. Enhanced cell attachment and osteoblastic activity by peptide-coated matrix in hydrogels. Biochem Biophys Res Commun (2003). , 15.

[18] Schilephake, H. Bone growth factors in maxillofacial skeletal reconstruction. Int J Oral Maxillofac Surg (2002). , 31(5), 469-84.

[19] Wikesjo, U. M, Huang, Y. H, Polimeni, G, & Qahash, M. Bone morphogenetic proteins: a realistic alternative to bone grafting for alveolar reconstruction. Oral Maxillofac Surg Clin North Am (2007). vi-vii., 19(4), 535-51.

[20] Marx, R. E, Carlson, E. R, Eichstaedt, R. M, Schimmele, S. R, Strauss, J. E, & Georgeff, K. R. Platelet-rich plasma: Growth factor enhancement for bone grafts. Oral Surg Oral Med Oral Pathol Oral Radiol Endod (1998). , 85(6), 638-46.

[21] Isidor, F. Influence of forces on peri-implant bone. Clin Oral Implants Res (2006). Suppl , 2, 8-18.

[22] Misch, C. Contemporary Implant Dentistry. Mosby Inc., Elsevier (2008). Third Edition., 200-229.

[23] Bidez, M. W, & Misch, C. E. Issues in bone mechanics related to oral implants. Implant Dent (1992)., 1(4), 289-94.

[24] Rieger, M. R, Adams, W. K, Kinzel, G. L, & Brose, M. O. Finite element analysis of bone-adapted and bone-bonded endosseous implants. J Prosthet Dent (1989)., 62(4), 436-40.

[25] Jivraj, S, & Chee, W. Treatment planning of implants in the aesthetic zone. Br Dent J (2006)., 201(2), 77-89.

[26] Marx, R. E, Shellenberger, T, Wimsatt, J, et al. Severely resorbed mandible: Predictable reconstruction with soft tissue matrix expansion (tent pole) grafts. J Oral Maxillofac Surg 60:8, (2002).

[27] Stevens, M. R, et al. Implant bone rings. One-stage three-dimensional bone transplant technique: a case report. J Oral Implantol, (2010)., 69-74.

Chapter 3

Inferior Alveolar Nerve Transpositioning for Implant Placement

Ali Hassani,
Mohammad Hosein Kalantar Motamedi and
Sarang Saadat

Additional information is available at the end of the chapter

1. Introduction

Premature loss of posterior teeth in the mandible, failure to replace lost teeth as well as systemic factors may result in progressive resorption of the alveolar ridge. At present, oral and maxillofacial surgeons aim to reconstruct the lost bone and masticatory function via posterior mandibular grafting and/or implants. However, anatomic limitations such as the inferior alveolar nerve (IAN) may limit this. Various treatment methods are available for treatment of patients with posterior mandibular atrophy presenting with a superficial IAN; each has its own merits and drawbacks. [1,2] Use of removable or fixed prosthetics and reconstruction of the dentoalveolar system by dental implants are among the available treatment options; a superficial IAN often precludes use of the latter. Implant-based reconstruction has several advantages i.e. allows for placement of longer implants, bone preservation, better functionality etc. and is gaining more proponents. However, certain conditions should be met in order for an implant to be placed. The most important condition is the quality and quantity of the bone. The amount of resorption, density of the bone and level of the nerve may limit implant placement. Reconstruction and rehabilitation of the dentoalveolar system in cases with alveolar ridge atrophy is a challenge for maxillofacial surgeons and prosthodontists. To date, several treatment options such as augmentation techniques with bone grafts [3], cartilage [4] or hydroxylapatite [5], vestibuloplasty [6] and several osteotomy techniques [7] have been suggested. Such treatments are still indicated as alternatives for cases in which for some reason dental implants cannot be placed [8]. In order to place an implant, we need adequate bone volume (both mediolaterally and mesiodistally) with optimal bone density.

This condition is usually not met in atrophic areas of the posterior mandible especially in patients that have been edentulous for some time. As the alveolar ridge becomes atrophied, the bony height from the crest of ridge to IAN decreases and the bone height in this area is often not enough to place an implant. Due to the increasing demand of patients for dental implants, strategies have been presented to overcome the obstacle of deficient alveolar bone height. These include guided bone regeneration (GBR), onlay bone graft, inter-positional sandwich bone graft, distraction osteogenesis (DO), all-on-four technique, use of short implants, lateral (or Lingual) positioning of implants and nerve transpositioning. Each of the aforementioned treatment options has its inherent advantages and disadvantages as well as indications and contraindications. In this chapter we discuss nerve transpositioning.

2. Nerve transpositioning

2.1. History

The first case of inferior alveolar nerve repositioning was reported by Alling in 1977 to rehabilitate patients with severe atrophy for dentures [9]. Jenson and Nock in 1987 carried out IAN transposition for placement of dental implants in posterior mandibular regions [10]. In 1992, Rosenquist performed the first case series study on 10 patients using 26 implants. He reported an implant survival rate of 96% for this procedure [11] and therefore, this technique was accepted as a treatment modality for reconstruction of the dentoalveolar system with dental implants in the posterior mandible. Consequently, research studies started to evaluate various surgical techniques developed for this procedure; their advantages, disadvantages, pitfalls and methods for preventing or decreasing complications were presented. As a result, this technique constantly improved. When looking at the history of different treatment modalities and surgical techniques in various academic fields we notice that most of them had limitations and complications at first but significantly improved with time and advancement of technology. Nerve transposition is a young procedure that needs further refinements in terms of technique and instrumentation to decrease complications.

2.2. Anatomy of the inferior alveolar nerve

The inferior alveolar nerve (IAN) is a branch of the mandibular nerve (V3) which is itself the third branch of the cranial nerve V (Figure 1). It runs downward on the medial aspect of the internal pterygoid muscle and passes inbetween the sphenomandibular ligament and the mandibular ramus entering through the mandibular foramen into the inferior alveolar canal innervating the teeth posterior to the mental foramen. At the mental foramen, the IAN divides into two branches namely the incisal and mental nerves (Figure 2). The incisal nerve is often described as the extension of the IAN innervating mandibular canines and incisors by passing through the bone [12].

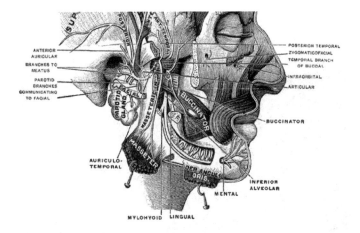

Figure 1. Inferior alveolar nerve path.

The inferior alveolar nerve gives off 3 branches inside the canal: Ramus Retromandibularis, Rami Molares or Molar Branch and Ramus Incisivus or Incisal Branch.

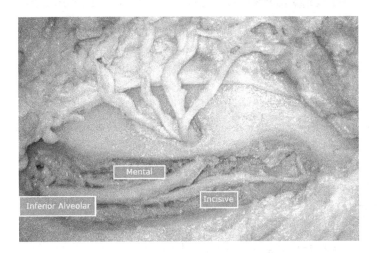

Figure 2. Branching of the inferior alveolar nerve into mental and incisive nerves at the mental foramen.

In some cases, the IAN canal is unilaterally or bilaterally bifid [13,14]. Thus, it is necessary to pay close attention to radiographic and CT examinations before nerve transposition in order to detect such cases and decrease the related risks (Figure 3).

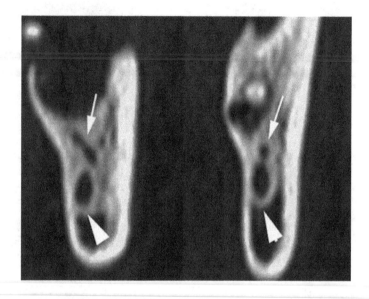

Figure 3. A coronal CT scan of a patient with a bifid mandibular nerve canal

2.2.1. Inferior alveolar nerve canal in edentulous patients

On panoramic radiographs of edentulous patients, the IAN canal in the body of the mandible is not very clear; thus, its path through the ramus and the opaque lines above and below the canal may not be clearly visible. Also, the closer we get to the mental foramen, the less visible the canal becomes [15,16]. Cesar et.al in their studies offered 2 types of classification for the IAN canal in edentulous patients. Vertically, the canal is located either in the upper or in the lower half of the mandible. In 73.7% of males and 70% of females the nerve is located in the lower half of the mandible (therefore, presence of the canal in the inferior half of the mandible is the most common occurrence). Branching of the IAN in edentulous patients falls into one of the following patterns: Type 1: Presence of one single trunk with no branching. Type 2: Presence of a series of separate nerve branches (most common type). Type 3: Presence of a molar plexus. Type 4: Presence of proximal and distal plexuses. Type 2 is the most prevalent pattern where a main trunk along with several single branches is directed towards the superior border of the mandible. The second most prevalent pattern is the presence of a small molar plexus at the proximal half of the IAN or Type 3 (Figure 4) [17].

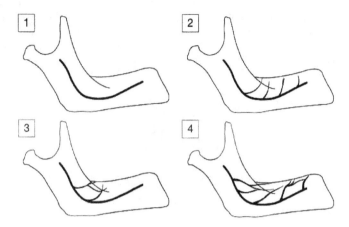

Figure 4. Variations of inferior alveolar nerve types in an edentulous mandible

2.2.2. The mental nerve

The mental nerve emerges at the mental foramen and divides beneath the depressor anguli oris muscle into 3 branches namely a descending branch that innervates the skin of the chin and 2 ascending branches innervating the skin and mucous membrane of the lower lip [13]. The patterns of emergence of the mental nerve at the mental foramen follows 1 of 3 patterns. Knowledge of these patterns is necessary for the surgeon before operating on this area. Type 1: The neurovascular bundle traverses anteriorly and then loops back to exit the mental foramen (anterior loop). Type 2: The nerve runs forward and exits the foramen along the canal path (absence of anterior loop). Type 3: The nerve exits the foramen perpendicular to the canal axis (absence of anterior loop). Type 1 is the most common pattern (61.5%) followed by type 2 (23.1%) and type 3 (15.4%) [18].

2.2.3. Contents of the mandibular canal and their location

Placing implants in areas adjacent to the IAN has increased significantly. Therefore, it is extremely important to know the contents of the canal and the exact location of components of the neurovascular bundle. According to histological examinations and MRI imaging, the inferior alveolar artery is located coronal to the nerve bundles inside the canal. Before entering the mandibular foramen, the artery is located inferior and posterior to the nerve. After entering the canal it changes its path at the mid length of the canal and runs superior and slightly medial to the nerve [18-20].The IAN usually has a round or oval cross section with a mean diameter of 2.2 mm. The mean diameter of the artery is 0.7 mm. The mean closest distance of the artery to a tooth apex is about 6 to 7 mm at the second molar area [20]. Yaghmaie et al. in 2011 confirmed the presence of lymphatic vessels in conjunction with the nerve trunks and blood vessels in all directions [21].The neurovascular bundle and its branches are responsi-

ble for sensation of pain, temperature, touch, pressure and proprioception of their innervat-
ed areas. The nerve is comprised of 1 or multiple fascicles. A collection of nerve fibers forms
a fascicle. Microscopic examination of neurovascular bundles usually shows 2 to 8 axon
bundles. Each fascicle contains about 500 to 1000 nerve fibers. Epineurium wraps around the
fascicles, protects them and contains blood vessels for nutrition (Figure 5) [18-20].

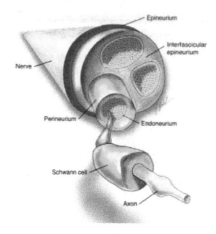

Figure 5. Schematic cross-section of the nerve. Nerve fascicles and fibers can be seen. Components in an orderly fashion from the outermost layer to the inner most include epineurium, perineurium, endoneurium and Schwann cells surrounding the axon.

2.2.4. Fascicular patterns

There are 3 fascicular patterns: The mono-fascicular pattern includes one big fascicle along
with perineurium and epineurium layers surrounding it (i.e. the facial nerve). The oligo-fascicular pattern includes 2 to 10 fascicles each covered by perineurium. Fascicles are intercon-
nected through the epineurium layer inbetween them; in this pattern, fascicles are usually of
the same size (nerve roots C6 and C7 have the oligo-fascicular pattern). The poly-fascicular
pattern includes more than 10 fascicles of various sizes i.e. inferior alveolar and lingual
nerves (Figure 6) [18-20].

As mentioned earlier, the IAN has a poly-fascicular pattern. The outer nerve fibers of the
bundle are called "mantle bundle". They usually innervate the proximal areas (molars). Following the administration of local anesthesia, this area is affected sooner and more efficiently since it is close to the side of the nerve bundle; whereas, core bundles innervate distal
areas (central and lateral) and are affected later and less efficiently by local anesthetics. Various senses are affected when administering local anesthetics depending on the nerve diameter and presence or absence of a myelin sheath. For instance, signal transmission is slower in
thinner non-myelinated nerve fibers. These fibers are affected more efficiently and more
quickly by the local anesthetics than large diameter, myelinated fibers that have faster signal

transmission. Non-myelinated fibers (sympathetic C fibers responsible for vascular tonicity and slow transmission of pain) and partially myelinated fibers (A delta fibers, fast transmission of pain) are affected sooner by the local anesthetics and also return to their normal state more quickly. On the contrary, thicker myelinated fibers (like A alpha and A Beta) that transmit deep sensations, pressure and proprioception are affected by local anesthetics later. In conclusion, general senses are affected clinically by the local anesthetics in the following order: First cold sensation through the autonomic nerves, then heat, pain, touch, pressure, vibration and eventually proprioception. Contents of the canal are responsible for innervation of dental pulps, periodontium, dental alveoli and soft tissues anterior to the mental foramen. Dental pulps receive unmyelinated sympathetic nerve fibers from the superior cervical trunk which enter the pulp accompanied by arterioles. Dental pulps also receive A delta myelinated sensory nerve fibers as well as unmyelinated nerve fibers (both from the trigeminal ganglion); together they form a large plexus below the odontoblastic layer in the pulp (Raschkow's plexus). In the Raschkow's plexus myelinated fibers lose their myelin sheath and penetrate into the odontoblastic layer. Today, they consider the phenomenon of fluid mobility inside the odontoblastic tubes (hydrodynamic theory) to be responsible for stimulation of nerve endings and sensing pain [12]. There are 2 aspects in the sensation of pain namely, a physiologic aspect and a psychological aspect which together create the unpleasant psycho-physiologic and complex experience of pain. From the physiologic point of view, stimulation of specific nerves (like A delta and C fibers) and transmission of the signal to the trigeminal ganglion is called "transduction". Passing over the signal from this site to upper centers (thalamus and cortex) is called "transmission" and "modulation". The three mentioned pathways comprise the physiologic aspect of pain that combined with the psychological aspect (previous experience, cultural behaviors, psychological state and medical status) create the unpleasant complex experience of pain [12].

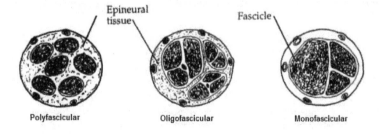

Figure 6. The three fascicular patterns. From right to left: Mono-fascicular, oligo-fascicular and poly-fascicular

2.2.5. Inferior alveolar nerve injury

Various factors can traumatize the IAN ranging from simple accidents like trauma from a needle during injection, bleeding around the nerve and even the local anesthetic drug itself, to maxillofacial traumas, pathologic lesions and surgical operations. Generally, the main nerve injuries are usually due to trauma or surgical operations among which, the most frequent ones are surgical extraction of mandibular third molars, endodontic treatment, implant placement, osteotomies (visor, sagittal, body of the mandible and subapical osteotomies), genioplasty, resection of mandibular cysts and tumors, partial mandibulectomy, fracture of the angle, ramus or body of the mandible, D.O. and IAN transpositioning. The nerve trunk is composed of 4 connective tissue sheaths. These membranes from the outermost to the innermost include mesoneurium, epineurium, perineurium and endoneurium. The mesoneurium suspends the nerve trunk within the soft tissue and contains vessels. The epineurium is a dense irregular connective tissue that protects the nerve against mechanical stress. The larger the epineurium (it usually measures 22 to 88% of the nerve diameter), the higher the nerve resistance against compressive forces compared to tensile forces. It should be mentioned that most nerve injuries are usually of a transient nature and will recover partially or completely. Epineural tissue wraps around nerve bundles and protects them against mechanical stress. Also, in many cases pressure due to severe inflammation or retention of fluid around the nerve trunk and subsequent development of transient ischemia in the epineurium cause clinical symptoms of neural dysfunction and disturbances. It is worth noting that the IAN is a poly-fascicular nerve. The smaller the number of nerve fascicles and the thicker the epineurium the more resistant the nerve is to pressure and vice versa (the greater the number of fascicles and the thinner the epineurium, the less resistant the nerves are towards pressure)[12,21-23]. It should be mentioned that poly-fascicular nerves like the IAN have a large number of small fascicles and therefore are more resistant to tensile forces compared to mono-fascicular or oligo-fascicular nerves [22].Perineurium wraps around the axon, Schwann cells and endoneurial sheath ; each nerve fiber is covered by the endoneurium sheath. Schwann cells are necessary for the axon to stay alive. They are the most sensitive cells to ischemia and radiation [12] (Figure 5).

2.2.6. Classification of nerve injury

There are 2 classifications available for nerve injury. The first was introduced by Seddon in 1943. He classified nerve injury into 3 types: Neuropraxia, Axonotmesis and Neurotmesis (from minor to major injury)[24]. The other classification was described by Sunderland [25] in 1987. He categorized 5 degrees of nerve injury : First degree where the axon and the covering sheath are intact. Epineural ischemia is probably the cause of the conduction block. Recovery is usually complete. Second degree where the axon is injured but endoneurium, perineurium and epineurium are intact. Recovery is often satisfactory. Third degree where the axon is injured but endoneurium is disrupted. However, of recovery. Fifth degree where there is complete transection with loss of continuity and less chance of spontaneous epineurium and perineurium are intact. Partial recovery may be achieved. Fourth degree where the axon, endoneurium and perineurium are all interrupted. However, epineurium is intact. There is a small chance recovery. Microscopic surgery is recommended (Table 1) [23].

Classification	Cause	Response	Recovery	Microscopic surgery
Neuropraxia(Sedd.) Grade 1 (Sunderland)	Compression, traction, small burn, acute infection	Neuritis, paresthesia, conduction block, no structural damage	Spontaneous recovery in less than 2 months	Not necessary unless a foreign body interrupts the process of nerve repair
Axonotmesis (Sedd.) Grade 2 (Sunder.)	Partial crushing, traction, burn, chemical trauma, hematoma, chronic infection	Intact epineurium, isolated axon loss, episodic dysesthesia	Spontaneous recovery within 2-4 months	Not indicated unless for decompression due to a foreign body or perineural fibrosis
Grade 3 (Sunder.)	Traction, crushing, contusion, burn, chemical trauma	Wallerian degeneration of axon, some internal fibrosis, peripheral pain	Poor sensory recovery, neuropathy for more than a year	Decompression and repair in case of poor function and continuous pain for 3 months
Grade 4 (Sunder.)	Complete crushing, severe traction, severe burn, direct chemical trauma	Neuroma-in-continuity, hypoesthesia, triggered hyperpathia	Permanent damage, minimal spontaneous recovery	Repair, resection of neuroma in case of unbearable pain after 3 months
Neurotmesis (Sedd.) Grade 5 (Sunder.)	Transverse incision on the nerve, laceration, laceration of the main nerve trunk	Neuroma at the site of incision, anesthesia, evolving deafferentation pain	Permanent damage, low spontaneous recovery	Resection of neuroma by neurorrhaphy or graft in case of poor function and lasting neuropathic pain

Table 1. Classification of nerve injury (Comparison of Sunderland and Seddon classifications)

2.2.7. Nerve changes following injury

Changes in central nervous system (CNS): The onset of such changes is 3-4 days or maximally 10-20 days after the injury. The neurons are in an anabolic state of protein synthesis. In humans, this can continue for years. The more proximal the location of injury, the higher the metabolic demand of the neuron. If the neuron is unable to supply such demand, cell death will occur. The best time for surgical repair when necessary is within 14 to 21 days after injury. After regeneration, the neuron gradually returns to its normal size and function.

Changes proximal to the site of injury: About an hour after trauma, a swelling develops within 1 cm proximal to the site of injury causing the area to enlarge up to 3 times its normal diameter. This swelling stays for a week or longer and then gradually subsides. On day 7, the proximal axon stump sprouts buds. These buds usually develop within a few millimeters distance from the site of injury from an intact node of Ranvier directed towards the distal end of the nerve. They cross the lesion on day 28, reconnect with the distal portion on day 42 and grow into it and advance (unless fibrous or scar tissue has formed). The more proximal the location of the injury, the longer it takes for a sprout to cross the lesion as the result of a more extensive inflammatory reaction.

Changes at the site of injury: During the next few hours after injury, proliferation of macrophages, perineural and epineural fibroblasts and Schwann cells occurs. On days 2 and 3, cell proliferation is seen proximal and distal to the site of injury. On day 7, Schwann cells play the major role. Fibrosis at the site of injury and imperfect positioning of regenerative fibers can result in formation of a neuroma.

Changes distal to the site of injury: Wallerian degeneration is the major characteristic of such changes in this area preparing the location for axonal sprouts budding out from the proximal stump. Death of all cellular components distal to the injury site is the key initiating event for Wallerian degeneration. On day 7 post-injury, the majority of cells at the distal portion disintegrate. This process is facilitated by the action of enzymes. By day 21, most cellular debris is engulfed and phagocytosed by Schwann cells. This cellular debridement is usually completed by day 42. Endoneurial tube becomes smaller, shrunken or even obstructed due to cell proliferation and excessive collagen formation. Its diameter is decreased by 50% after 3 months and only 10 to 25% of its primary diameter may be left open after 12 months. This phenomenon is called distal atrophy when the entire nerve trunk distal to the site of injury is shrunken and atrophied. Tubules formed by Schwann cells and surrounded by collagen guide the sprouts distally. Although the number of sprouts is various and may be up to 4 times the normal number, during regeneration volume and number of sprouts decrease and the final number will end up to be smaller than the original number and the diameter of the new axon will be smaller as well. When a sprout reaches the distal tube, the metabolic activity of the Schwann cells increases again and myelin is reproduced by the Schwann cells. However, the quality of the newly formed myelin is not as good as the quality of the primary myelin. The new axon has a smaller diameter and is placed in thinner endoneurial tubes. The new myelin is not similar to the old one. The nodes of Ranvier are shorter and therefore cause a decrease in nerve conduction velocity in this area. Axon regeneration speed is different in various circumstances but it is on average 1 to 3 mm a day.

Changes in the target organ: At the target sensory organ, receptors suffer from progressive deformities but following reinnervation even after several years the target organ will have no sensory impairment or disturbances. For skin flaps as well, reinnervation resumes pain, temperature and touch sensations perfectly. For target motor organs however, reinnervation of the respected muscle does not occur even 12 months after nerve transection. This is not because of changes in neuromuscular junction end plate but probably due to irreversible interstitial fibrosis in muscle fibers [13].

Clinical examination of sensory impairment of the lower lip following IAN injury:

Before discussing the clinical examinations, we explain the definition of common clinical terms (Table 2).

Anesthesia	Absence of any sensation
Paresthesia	Abnormal sensation even spontaneously or for no reason
Analgesia	No pain in response to a normally painful stimulus
Dysesthesia	An unpleasant abnormal sensation that can be spontaneous or for a reason
Hyperalgesia	Hypersensitivity to harmful stimuli
Hyperesthesia	Hypersensitivity to all stimuli except for special senses
Hypoalgesia	Decreased sensitivity to stimuli
Hypoesthesia	Decreased sensitivity to all stimuli except for special senses
Allodynia	Pain due to a stimulus that does not normally cause pain
Neuralgia	Pain that is distributed in one or several nerve fibers
Deafferentation pain	Pain due to decreased sensory afferents into the CNS
Neuropathic pain	Pain due to a primary lesion or nervous system dysfunction
Causalgia	Burning pain immediately or several months after injury
Anesthesia dolorosa	Pain felt in an area which is completely numb to touch
Synesthesia	Stimulation of one sensory or cognitive pathway leads to experience in a second cognitive or sensory pathway due to misdirected axonal buds resulting in misperception of the location of touch or pain
Central pain	Pain due to a primary lesion or central nervous system dysfunction
Hyperpathia	A painful syndrome characterized by hyper-responsiveness to a stimulus. Hyperpathia may be associated with hyperesthesia, hyperalgesia or dysesthesia

Table 2. Frequently used terms during clinical examination of neurosensory disturbances

2.2.8. Clinical tests

Static light touch: For this test a bunch of nylon filaments with same length and different thickness mounted on a plastic handle is used. The patient closes his eyes and says "yes" whenever he feels a light touch to the face and points to the exact spot where he felt the touch. Brush directional discrimination: For this test, the finest nylon filaments from the previous test or a brush with more filaments are used. The patient states if any sensation is detected and in which direction the filament or brush moved. **Two point discrimination**: In this test the distance between two points is altered. With the patient's eyes closed the test is initiated with the points essentially touching so that the patient is able to discriminate only one point. **Pin pressure nociception**: For this test the most common instrument is the algesimeter which is a simple instrument made from a no.4 Taylor needle and an orthodontic strain gauge. The sharp point of the needle is used to test nociception and the blunt end to test for pressure detection and hyperpathia. The needle is placed vertically on the skin. The pressure is increased every few seconds until the patient feels the sharpness (usually with 15 to 25 g) and then the needle is gently removed. The same is done for the affected area as well. No response to pin pressure up to 100 g is defined as anesthesia. An exaggerated response to pin pressure relative to an unaffected area is defined as hyperalgesia and a reduced response to touch relative to an unaffected area is considered as hypoalgesia. **Thermal discrimination**: This is an adjuvant test and is not es-

sential. Minnesota Thermal Disks are the most common instruments used for this assessment. Ice, ethyl chloride spray, acetone, and water are also used. The simplest method is
to use an applicator dipped into acetone or ethyl chloride. When pain is a symptom of
nerve injury, diagnostic nerve blocks using local anesthesia can be very helpful in decid-
ing whether or not micro-reconstructive surgery is indicated. It is important to start with
low concentrations of anesthetic drug. Injections should be performed starting from the
periphery towards the center to ease the pain. If the pain is not alleviated there is a
chance that collateral sprouts from the other side are present. If the persisting pain is aggravated by cold, is spontaneous, and of burning type and long lasting, then allodynia,
hyperpathia, causalgia and sympathetic pain should considered in the differential diagnosis. In such cases, diagnostic stellate ganglion block is helpful in differentiating causalgia
from sympathetic pain [10,12,24]. There are various causes of pain following traumatic
nerve injury including nerve compression, neuroma, anesthesia dolorosa, causalgia and
sympathetic pain, central pain and deafferentation, nerve laceration, nerve ischemia and
chemical stimulation.

Clinical and radiographic evaluation. For clinical assessment of a patient who is a candidate for dental implants and suffers from atrophic mandibular alveolar ridge should first
prepare study casts and then the occlusal relationship should be recorded. The following
points should also be considered:

The area of the edentulous atrophic alveolar ridge: If the edentulous area extends interi-
orly up to the canine the surgeon should consider mental nerve transpositioning.[1]. In
edentulous patients, absence of incisal sensation following nerve distalization does not
cause problems but in patients with incisal teeth this can result in an unpleasant sensation
in the anterior segment which is usually described as a sense of dullness in these teeth.
The distance between the occlusal surface of maxillary teeth and mandibular alveolar
ridge. In some cases, despite alveolar ridge resorption there is not enough space between
the occlusal surface of the maxillary teeth and the mandibular ridge which is required for
placing the implant prosthesis. It is usually due to the patient's previous occlusion (mainly in deep bite cases) or over-eruption of the opposing teeth. Augmentative methods often
cannot be used (Figure 7]. In such cases, the only available option seems to be nerve
transpositioning [3,22,26].

**Evaluation of the relationship between the mandibular alveolar ridge and maxillary al-
veolar ridge in the horizontal plane:** The necessity of lateral augmentation simultaneous
with nerve transposition or vertical augmentation should also be evaluated by clinical examination and study of the patient's casts.

Radiographic evaluation: Every patient who is a candidate for nerve transposition is required to obtain panoramic radiography and CBCT scans (Figure 7).

The length of bone above the canal, anomalies, distance of the canal from the buccal cortex
and also thickness of the cortex for ostectomy are all evaluated on panoramic radiography.
Exact location and precise anatomy of the mental foramen and anterior loop can also be
evaluated [27]. In rare cases, the IAN canal may be completely attached to the medial or lat-

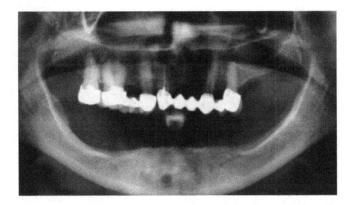

Figure 7. Panoramic radiography of an atrophic posterior mandible. Note the inadequate length of bone over the canal for implant placement.

eral cortex on CBCT. In such cases, implants can be easily placed buccally or lingually to the canal with no need for extensive surgery. Additionally, by analysis and reconstruction of scanned images using CAD-CAM, it is feasible to determine the path of the canal and place the implants in atrophic areas.

2.3. Indications, contraindications and limitations

Babbush mentioned several indications for nerve transpositioning; namely placement of removable prosthetics, stabilizing the remaining anterior teeth, stabilizing the temporomandibular joint, and establishing muscular balance following reconstruction of the dentoalveolar system. He also discussed some related limitations. This procedure is technically difficult and requires adequate expertise. The surgeon should have adequate experience, sufficient anatomical knowledge and necessary skills to fully manage peri-operative and post-operative complications. Accordingly, the most significant risk of surgery is nerve injury due to surgical manipulations and the surgical procedure itself. Although rare, mandibular fracture should also be considered as a risk factor especially in cases with severe mandibular atrophy (Figure 8) [28].

Resenquise et al. in their studies on nerve transpositioning procedure mentioned the following indications and contraindications for this operation:

Indications: Less than 10-11 mm bone height above the canal, when the quality of the spongy bone does not provide sufficient stability for implant placement

Contraindications: Height of bone over the canal is less than 3 mm. The patient has thick cortical bone buccally and thin neurovascular bundle. The patient is susceptible to infection or bleeding. Limitation in accessing the surgical site [9-11,29,30]

According to author's personal experience, nerve transpositioning in cases where the bone height over the canal is less than 3 mm is still feasible. We can transpose the nerve from the

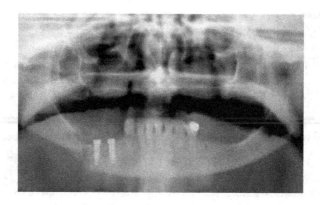

Figure 8. Mandibular fracture in a patient with severe mandibular atrophy following nerve transpositioning.

alveolar crest laterally, and after placing the implant with bone graft material. More details in this regard will be discussed subsequently.

2.4. Surgical procedure of nerve transpositioning

Pre-operative consultation: Before choosing nerve transpositioning, we should first scrutinize the required criteria. According to the literature, 100% of patients who undergo nerve transposition develop various degrees of sensory nerve dysfunction of the lips. Therefore, the patient and his/her family members should be well informed relevant to the phases of treatment, duration of surgery, post-operative general complications and most importantly provided with knowledge about the post-operative lip paresthesia which will definitely occur and may last for up to 6 months and in some cases it lasts longer or is very severe may require microscopic surgery [10,31-33]. Despite the above mentioned explanations, the patient may not fully comprehend what paresthesia actually feels like. In such cases, we recommend performing an inferior alveolar nerve block for the patient using bupivacaine for anesthesia so that the patient can experience anesthesia and paresthesia for 8 to 12 hours. We should also explain the advantages of this treatment modality for the patient including shorter treatment duration, no need for autogenous bone grafts and no donor site morbidity, minimum use of bone replacement material and obviating the need for additional surgery [9,10,33].

2.4.1. Technique

Inferior alveolar nerve transpositioning for implant placement is usually performed by 2 techniques: **IAN transpositioning without mental nerve transpositioning or involvement of mental foramen:** This is usually employed when the edentulous area and alveolar ridge resorption does not include the premolars. This technique has been called nerve lateralization in some articles (Figure 9-12 A). **IAN transpositioning with mental nerve transpositioning or involvement of mental foramen:** In cases where the edentulous area and ridge resorption include the premolar teeth: there is a need for transpositioning of mental neuro-vascular bundle and even transection of incisal nerve and transposing the nerve distally (associated with mental nerve and mental foramen involvement). This method has also been called nerve distalization by some [1,9,28,34] (Figure 12 B).

Phases of surgery: Nerve transpositioning can be performed under local anesthesia alone, local anesthesia along with sedation or under general anesthesia based on the patient's condition. Local anesthesia includes inferior alveolar nerve block plus local infiltrating anesthesia in the form of lidocaine plus vasoconstrictor at the buccal mucosa. 1-Incision is made on the alveolar crest starting from the anterior border of the ramus forward. At the mesial surface of the mandibular canine a releasing incision is made anteriorly and towards the vestibular sulcus in order to avoid injuring mental nerve branches. In cases where the treatment plan includes placement of dental implants in the same surgical step, soft tissue incision should be made in a way that part of keratinized gingiva is placed in the buccal and part of it on the lingual side of the healing abutment (Figures 10 and 11) [1,31-35].

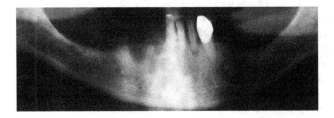

Figure 9. A patient with edentulous posterior mandibular region along with bone resorption who is a candidate for nerve transposition surgery.

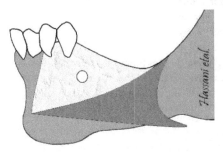

Figure 10. Flap design: An incision is made on the alveolar crest along with a releasing incision at the mesial of mandibular canine.

2-Retracting the mucoperiosteal flap is done so that the mental foramen is totally exposed and the dissection is extended towards the inferior border. Considering the radiographic and CBCT evaluations along with the fact that the neurovascular canal is usually located 2 mm below the mental foramen, it is necessary to expose the lateral surface of the body of the mandible and release the periosteum around the mental nerve (Figure 10) [1,36]. 3-Bone removal on the lateral surface of the canal is done while preserving the maximum thickness of buccal bone as this especially important. Presence of adequate bone thickness in this area results in better and faster healing of the bone defect adjacent to the implant where nerve transposition has been performed. Bone can be removed using a diamond round bur or piezosurgery device [1,6].

In the first technique which is usually performed for treatments other than dental implants a piece of bone is removed as a block and then the canal is exposed. This method can be indicated for simultaneous implant surgery when there is adequate bone height over the canal. In such cases, even after resecting a bone block, a sufficient amount of bone still remains at the lateral side of the implant [26]. Rosenquist reported that in this method, it is difficult to maintain a proper angulation when placing the implant because a great extent of buccal bone has been removed for nerve transposition and accessing the canal [30]. In patients who are candidates for implants, cortical bone preferably should not be removed as a block because in such patients there is limited amount of bone available in the superior and lateral sides of the canal which should be preserved. If the surgical technique does not include manipulation of the mental nerve, bone is removed using a round bur number 700 or 701, a straight handpiece and copious normal saline for irrigation or a piezosurgery device. Bone removal is initiated 3-4 mm distal to the mental foramen and follows the canal path posteriorly and superiorly. Bone removal should extend 4-6 mm posterior to the intended location of the last implant. We should try to remove the smallest amount of bone possible from the buccal cortex. Excessive bone removal along with extensive drilling for implant placement can result in temporary mandibular weakening followed by increased risk of mandibular fracture which has been reported in the literature. Bone preservation helps in primary and final implant stability and shortens the recovery time. After removing the cortical bone, a curette may be used for removal of spongy bone and cortical layer of the canal in cases where the cortical layer surrounding the canal is not dense or thick. A special instrument (Hassani nerve protector) is required to protect the nerve while the cortical layer has to be removed using surgical burs or piezosurgery device. Bone removal in close vicinity to the neurovascular bundle should be performed patiently and thoroughly. This is usually performed using special curettes parallel to the surface of nerve bundles in an antero-posterior direction. Tiny bone spicules around the nerve should be removed. The area should be thoroughly irrigated so that the nerve bundle can be clearly seen (Figure 11 A - D) [1,2,4,9,10].

Another method that has been suggested is drilling the bone surrounding the canal using a hand piece and a round bur. The surgeon carefully enters a probe (round end with no sharp edge) into the canal through the mental foramen and determines the canal path. Then according to this test and after evaluating the canal path on the radiographs, the surgeon inserts the tip of the nerve protector into the canal. This instrument has been designed, patented and manufactured by the author (Hassani nerve protector). This instrument should be placed in between the nerve and the bone in order to protect the nerve. The buccal bone is drilled using a bur. By directing the bur distally, the nerve protector is also moved distally inbetween the nerve and bone to protect the nerve at all times. The bone chips are collected

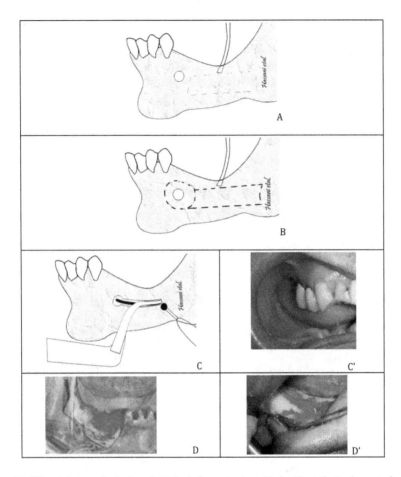

Figure 11. Different designs of osteotomy A: Method of removing bone block without the involvement of mental foramen: In this technique, a bur is used to outline the location of bone block on mandibular buccal cortex by a distance from the inferior border of mandible and alveolar crest. The mesial incision should be made in 3-4 mm away from the mental foramen. Then the buccal bone surrounding the canal is removed carefully by reciprocal motion using an osteotome (Chisel). The remaining spongy bone around the canal is collected while protecting the nerve and stored for bone grafting. At this time the nerve is exposed. This method is associated with the risk of losing the buccal bone. B: Removal of bone block along with mental foramen involvement: Similar to the previous method, a bur is used to outline the bone block area. An osteotome (chisel) is used to remove the bone block and the spongy bone is removed using a curette. In this technique, the preparation design includes the surroundings of the mental foramen. While keeping an adequate distance from mental foramen a circle is drawn with the center being the foramen using a round bur and the cortical bone is resected. By doing so, we have 2 bone blocks one posterior to the mental foramen and the other one around it through which the nerve has passed. This mesial segment with the nerve passing through it is put aside with great caution and when operation is over it is put back in its original location. This technique is indicated when the edentulous atrophic area has extended and involved the premolar area and there is a need for replacing the lost premolar teeth. This method carries the risk of incisal nerve transection by the surgeon. This method has been called nerve distalization. C-D: Oral views.

by a bone collector in the process. In this technique, while the nerve is protected minimum amount of bone is removed from the buccal cortex and the maximum amount of bone is preserved in an atrophic ridge for implant placement which results in maximum primary stability of the implant. Also, mandibular bone weakening is minimal in this method which is a great advantage of this technique. The neurovascular bundle inside the canal is freed using special curettes and is moved laterally using a nerve hook (Figure 12). Then a 10 mm wide gauze cord or elastic band is passed below it retracting the nerve away from the surgical site decreasing ischemic trauma to the nerve. It also retracts the nerve away from the surgical site during the operation reducing the risk of nerve damage (Figure 13) [9,34,24,35].

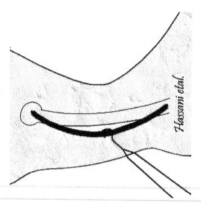

Figure 12. Spongy bone surrounding the nerve is removed using a spoon shaped curette. The nerve is released and slowly retracted from the canal using a nerve hook. The hook should be rounded at the end and polished.

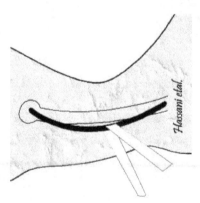

Figure 13. The nerve is retracted from the site using a gauze band 10 mm wide or elastic band in order to protect it from any damage during implant placement. The advantage of elastic band is that if it is pulled during surgery the traction is neutralized by the band and not transferred to the nerve.

Some studies recommend piezosurgery for bone removal in nerve transposition surgery. This device causes vibrations in the range of 20-200 micrometers and cuts through the mineralized tissue completely and smoothly. If soft tissue or the neurovascular bundle comes in contact with this device it stops to function because the device is made in a way that it stops working when it is in contact with unmineralized tissue. This device is especially beneficial when a small osteotomy is going to be performed [9]. Among the disadvantages of this device we can mention the long duration of time that it takes to remove bone. Also, there is still controversy regarding the indications of this device and some believe that vibrations may damage the nerve. Further investigations are required regarding indications of using this device in nerve transposition surgery [9,10].

Preparing the implant placement site and implant positioning: In this phase, the mucoperiosteal flap and nerve are raised and the surgeon starts drilling. The implant should be long enough to pass the canal and engage the basal below the canal to achieve sufficient primary stability. Then, the implant is inserted (Figures 14 and 15) [1,9,31].

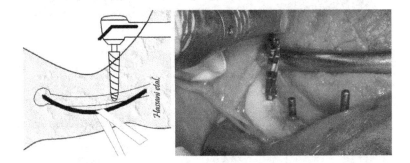

Figure 14. Cavity preparation and bone drilling when the nerve is retracted from the site using a umbilical tape 10 mm wide or elastic band in order to protect it from any damage during drilling or implant placement.(Surgical Drill, Dentium Co.)

Repositioning the neurovascular bundle inside the canal: Before this phase, the surgeon should decide whether or not to place materials between the implant and the nerve. There is a lot of controversy in this regard and some studies have been performed on animal models in this respect. In a study by Yoshimoto et al. on rabbits, no difference was observed microscopically after placing and not placing a membrane between the implant and the nerve bundle [37]. However, on animal model studies clinical signs and symptoms of nerve stimulation cannot be assessed and only microscopic evaluation is feasible. The author's preference is to place a collagen membrane or bone material in between the implant and nerve. A potential advantage of bone over a membrane is that if proper healing occurs in the area, the contact area of implant and bone will increase (Figure 16). Before releasing the nerve from the elastic band, the mentioned material must be inserted in between the nerve and implant. This way the nerve will be in a vent that is adjacent to implants medially and covered by the mucoperiosteal flap. Alternatively, the nerve may be left to lie passively outside of the canal.

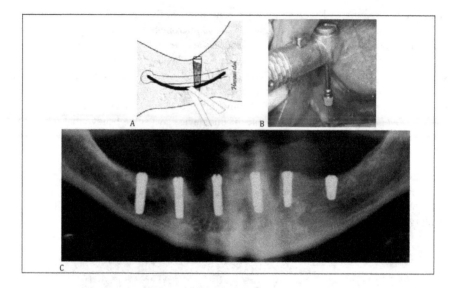

Figure 15. A-C: Implant is placed into the bone. Implant can be seen by the surgeon in part of its insertion path when passing the empty nerve canal. Therefore, the surgeon can insert the implant a few centimeters below the canal into the basal bone and benefit from the advantages of a bicortical implant such as adequate primary stability and shorter recovery time.(Implantium Implants,Dentium Co.)

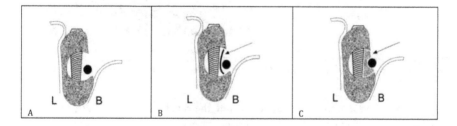

Figure 16. Replacing the nerve inside the canal and different viewpoints in this regard: A: Some believe that there is no need for placing a membrane or any material to prevent contact of implant and nerve. The nerve is placed inside the canal alone. B: Some believe that it is necessary to place a membrane (arrow) between the implant and the nerve to prevent risk of sensory disturbances in the future. C: Inserting bone dust (arrow) collected by bone collector between the implant and nerve (based on the author's experience this way the nerve is not in direct contact with the implant and bone dusts also enhances the process of bone regeneration and repair resulting in formation of more bone around the implant). Alloplast or xenograft bone powder may also be used.

Suturing and closing the wound: The decision to submerge the implant using a cover screw or using a healing abutment for single phase implant surgery should be made based on the condition of surgical site, presence of adequate amount of bone at alveolar crest and type of implant used. The surgical wound is then sutured (Figure 17 and 18).

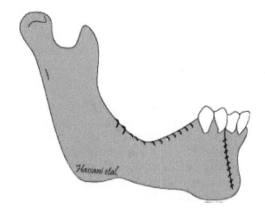

Figure 17. Gingival flap is put back in its location and sutured.

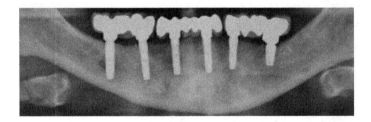

Figure 18. Same patient in Figure 16; Two years after loading the implants. Note the bone level. (Implantium Implants, Dentium Co.)

In patients with an atrophic alveolar ridge involving the premolar area or those with an edentulous mandibular ridge along with alveolar crest atrophy who need implant placement IAN transposition in the posterior mandible and mental nerve transposition is also necessary most of the time. This transposition is usually associated with incisal nerve transection. In such cases, the patients will not have any problems related to incisal nerve transection but in cases where transposition of the nerve is intended and the patient has vital anterior mandibular teeth, nerve transection may result in patient having an unpleasant sensation in these teeth. In some cases, even root canal therapy may be required. However, several studies have reported that no problems related to anterior mandibular teeth were seen [1,9,35].

Sectioning the incisal branch of the inferior alveolar nerve, releasing the neurovascular bundle and moving it backwards in order to avoid traction is called nerve distalization [9]. Based on the author's experience, in many cases it is possible to transpose the mental nerve without sectioning the incisal nerve. In the method of nerve transposition without releasing the mental nerve, great traction force is exerted on the nerve when keeping it out of the surgical site. According to the literature, the highest number of nerve injuries occurs during anterior osteotomy because the nerve trunk becomes thinner at mental foramen and is therefore more susceptible to injury. That is why nerve transposition without involving the mental foramen has the least sensory complications and side effects. According to the literature, by preserving 3-4 mm bone distal to the mental foramen during nerve transposition we can reduce inferior alveolar nerve damage because the nerve is thinner and more susceptible to injury at this specific location [32].

Vasconcelos et al. believes that at least 5 mm bone height above the canal is necessary in case selection for nerve transposition whereas, Kahnberg and colleagues believe that 2 to 3 mm bone thickness above the canal is adequate [9,10]. In cases where minimum requirement of bone height above the canal does not exist some authors suggest to do a bone graft before nerve transposition and implant placement [9]. However, fixing the grafts especially blocks of autogenous bone to the limited remaining bone above the canal is difficult and is associated with a risk of nerve injury by the screws. Based on the author's experience in such cases we can transpose the nerve from the alveolar crest laterally. Bone is removed from the alveolar crest, and when the nerve is exposed we move it upward and outward and start drilling for implant placement from inside the canal while the nerve is retracted laterally from the buccal cortex. Bone graft is placed inside the canal anterior and posterior to the implant. The nerve is placed into a newly formed groove from the posterior area of the last implant (Figure 19).

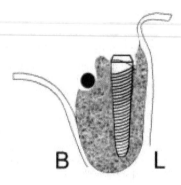

Figure 19. The IAN is located at the alveolar crest following ridge atrophy. The nerve is removed from the crest, implant hole is prepared from inside the canal, the implant is positioned and finally the nerve is repositioned in the lateral cortex of the mandible.

Histological findings associated with nerve transposition and implant placement. Yoshimoto and colleagues evaluated the condition of tissues surrounding the implant 8 weeks after nerve transposition surgery and simultaneous implant placement; they observed that none of the implants were exposed and all were perfectly stable. No infection or inflammation was observed at the site. In all cases bone formation between the implant and neurovascular bundle was observed and no direct contact was seen between them.

Research demonstrates that bone formation around the implant surface sand blasted with aluminum oxide was 2.5 times greater than a smooth titanium surface. Bone formation around the neurovascular bundle prevents the implant from having direct physical contact with the bundle and therefore the nerve structure will be protected from mechanical or thermal trauma. Microscopic sections show the formation of a vascular network in the adjacent tissues which proves that there is no need for placing a barrier or any kind of graft material to separate the nerve from the implant [35].

In Kahnberg et al. study on a dog, healing was not complete after 14 weeks but none of the implants were exposed. Histological examination showed that in cases where membrane had not been placed a small contact was present between the nerve bundle and the implant. Plasma cells, macrophages, polymorphonuclears, and granulocytes were alternately seen next to the membrane. Several giant cells and macrophages were also seen. Vascular buds were seen where membrane had been placed (compared to areas where no membrane had been used). In some cases, a capsule with less than 10 μm thickness was seen in some areas between the implant and the nerve. When membrane is used the distance between the nerve bundle and the implant will be 4 to 8 times greater. The mean distance between the implant and the nerve was 348.3 μm when using a membrane and 39.8 μm when not using it. There is no contact between the nerve and the implant when using a membrane but the bone was not seen around the implant either [38].

2.5. Important considerations in nerve transposition surgery

2.5.1. Patient selection

The surgical process is complicated and occurrence of sensory disturbances is definite. Therefore, the surgeon should evaluate the patient's mental condition. Some people are stressed out and over sensitive even towards the smallest surgical complications. Such patients do not have tolerance and compatibility skills and therefore are not good candidates for nerve transposition surgery. Providing data and acquainting the patient with phases of surgery and probable complications: Thorough explanation should be provided for the patient in an understandable and comprehendible manner regarding surgical and neural complications. The sense of anesthesia that may occur should be well described for the patient and it also should be mentioned that the anesthesia may be permanent and irreversible.

1. CBCT should be obtained for precise evaluation of the canal and bone thickness around it.

2. Dexamethasone should be administered before the surgery

3. The surgeon should have full knowledge regarding anatomy and physiopathology of nerve injury and be able to evaluate the clinical course of nerve dysfunction after the surgery.

4. The surgeon's skill and expertise are very important and magnification loops should be used.

5. Delicate instruments required for this type of surgery should be available (for minimal injury). Also, the surgeon should have the knowledge and skills for repairing the nerve in case serious damage is done to the nerve during surgery.

6. In cases where the canal is located in the center or lingually on CBCT, the surgeon should expect a more complex surgery.

7. In cases where the nerve transposition surgery extends further posterior and involves the 2nd molar area, the surgery can be more complicated due to the thicker cortical bone and limited access to the area.

8. Using low level laser after surgery reduces the inflammation and improves recovery.

9. The surgeon should be familiar with and have adequate skills regarding nerve reconstruction surgery and the instruments required for it.

2.5.2. Post-operative measures

Antibiotic therapy and administration of analgesics and NSAIDs post-operatively are similar to that of implant surgery and there are no specific recommendations in this regard in the literature. Antibiotic and corticosteroid prophylaxis is recommended because of the extensiveness and duration of surgery. Using corticosteroids pre- and post-operatively helps in decreasing the symptoms. However, there is no consensus in this regard but since inflammation can be among the causes of nerve dysfunction, corticosteroid therapy can be beneficial.

The most common sensory complications following nerve transposition are hypoesthesia, paresthesia and hyperesthesia. The most common causes of nerve dysfunction include the mechanical trauma to the nerve and ischemia following extracting the bundle from the canal, nerve traction during surgery, edema and probable hematoma and or chronic compression after the surgery [9,10]. According to Hirsch and Branemark, the main cause of sensory disturbances is nutritional impairment of the nerve due to injury to the microvascular circulation of nerve fibers as the result of mechanical trauma. Thermal and pain sensation nerve fibers are more resistant to compressive traumatic forces and ischemia than larger fibers responsible for touch sensation [1]. Therefore, great attention should be paid during and after surgery to minimize the factors responsible for ischemia and mechanical trauma such as;

1. Avoiding exerting too much traction upon the nerve and when lateralizing the nerve and during nerve transposition, try to transform the contact point to a contact area.

2. During ostectomy care must be taken not to injure the nerve with rotary instruments, curette or elevator. When removing the bone cortex over the nerve, the author recommends using the nerve protector designed specifically for this purpose by the author himself; it fits inside the nerve canal over the nerve (Figure12 C and D'). Direct contact of rotary or other surgical instruments with the nerve is among the most serious injuries in this type of surgery.

3. In order to lateralize the nerve, use instruments with minimal traction and prevent ischemia to the nerve. Instruments that have large contact area with the nerve and mini-

mum thickness are preferred to be placed between the nerve and the location of drilling for implant placement.

4. The retracted bundle should be constantly moistened by normal saline.

5. Prevent development of hematoma because it applies pressure on the nerve trunk.

6. After inserting the implant, autogenous bone powder or collagen membrane should be placed between the implant and the nerve bundle (as discussed earlier).

7. Use of anti-inflammatory drugs before and after surgery: Some articles have recommended administration of corticosteroids pre- and post-operatively or high dose ibuprofen 800 mg TDS for 3 weeks [39].

8. Using vitamin B complex supplements (studies have shown that B complex and vitamin E supplementation improves nerve function and decreases neuropathy. Vitamin B family especially B1 and B12 can prevent nerve injury and improve natural growth of the nerve by preserving and protecting the lipid-rich covering of nerve terminals. Alcohol consumption causes vitamin B deficiency and therefore should be avoided [40].

9. Use of low level laser (LLL) immediately after surgery 4 times a week for 10 sessions. Studies suggest using LLL as a non-invasive non-surgical method for faster recovery from paresthesia may obviate the need for surgery in nerve injuries. Use of GaA1As laser causes the patient's subjective and objective symptoms to disappear. Low level laser increases nerve function and capacity of myelin production [10,41]. Bleeding inside the canal can cause a hematoma or compartment syndrome [42]. The incidence of post-operative neuropraxia, permanent anesthesia and paresthesia decreases when only the thicker parts of the neurovascular bundle are manipulated compared to the manipulation of thinner parts or terminal branches. Therefore, although nerve transposition in more posterior areas like the 2nd molar area is technically more complex, it is usually associated with smaller risk of serious and long term injuries to the nerve because the neurovascular bundle is thicker in this region. Regeneration process of nerve following mild compression or crushing takes several weeks to 6 months [10]. If recovery does not occur in this time period, we should consider the possibility of permanent anesthesia. Some researchers believe that sensory changes following implant placement and nerve transposition should be considered as a normal consequence of treatment and not a sequel or complication [10,43].

2.5.3. Pharmaceutical therapy and treatment of traumatic nerve injuries

Course of nerve recovery and symptoms vary based on the type and severity of the primary injury. In most cases, only time and regular patient visits are required. Other cases may need drug therapy or microscopic reconstructive neural surgery (**Algorithm 1**). In case of nerve transection, we can suture the free ends without traction but primary and simultaneous graft should never be performed. If the nerve is under traction, greater fibrosis will develop at the site of repair. In cases with nerve compression or traction, the surgeon should release the nerve and eliminate the traction or compression and prevent ischemia due to mechanical

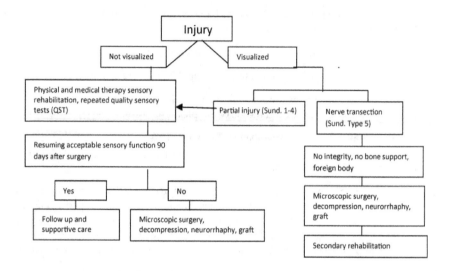

Algorithm 1. How to decide about the treatment and management of inferior alveolar nerve injury

trauma [12]. After nerve repair, clinical tests should be performed weekly during the first month and then monthly for 5 months. It is especially important to do the test in the first month to diagnose if neuroma or neuropathic pains develop [39]. In case of presence of neuropathic pains, primary management includes nerve block by local anesthetics, use of analgesics and nerve stimulation through the skin (30 min a day for 3 weeks). If post traumatic neural pains do not alleviate pain after 3-4 weeks, administration of various drugs have been recommended [12].

Some of the medications used for neuropathic pain control:

1. Fluphenazine 1 mg, 3 times a day along with Amitriptyline 75 mg before bedtime

2. Doxepin (tricylic antidepressant) 25 mg 3 times a day

3. Carbamazepine up to 100 mg/day

4. Baclofen up to 80 mg/day

5. For sympathetical pain we can do injections for stellate ganglion block. Alpha 2 adrenergic blockers (clonidine 0.1 to 0.3 mg/day based on tolerance) 5 times a week for 3 weeks; sympathectomy can also be used.

6. In case of acute pains fast-acting anticonvulsants (like clonazepam) 2 to 10 mg/day may be useful.

7. Titrated Gabapentin anticonvulsant 600 to 3000 mg is beneficial for chronic pains following traumatic injuries. If the patient also suffers from sleep disorders, antidepressants may be used at bedtime.

8. Anti-inflammatory drugs, analgesics, anti-anxiety medications and sleeping pills can also be used in addition to the above mentioned medications.

9. Topical lidocaine gel (for mucus membrane) and 5% lidocaine patches (for skin) which are released slowly within 12 hours are used for the mucous membrane and skin of the irritated areas or trigger zones.

10. Intravenous injection of lidocaine may be used sometimes for diagnostic purposes. In such cases, first normal saline is injected as a placebo and then the patient's symptoms are evaluated and then 1 mg/kg lidocaine is slowly injected intravenously within 2 minutes and the patient is asked about its effects every 30 seconds. Pain relief (more than 30%) indicates the effectiveness of intravenous lidocaine injection which shows the neuropathic origin of the pain and we should consider the probable efficacy of medications with central effects such as anticonvulsants [12, 22].

Nerve reconstruction

In case of requiring inferior alveolar nerve reconstructive surgery, it is important to maintain the integrity of the nerve. First, the nerve is exposed and the surrounding tissues are released so that the extensiveness of injury is evident. Compression injuries result in development of fibrosis. In such cases, first lactate ringer's solution is subcutaneously injected in the fibrotic area with a 30 gauge needle to separate the epineurium from the fascicles and determine the extension of fibrous tissue. Then the fibrous tissue is eliminated by a fine longitudinal incision over the epineurium. If the fibrous tissue is extensive and has penetrated into the fascicles we have to dissect this area and suture the free ends of the nerve together. Inferior alveolar nerve is usually composed of 12 to 30 small fascicles with scattered epineurium wrapped around them. Therefore, extensive fibrosis between the fascicles rarely occurs unless in case of major injury. If there is a neuroma, similar to extensive fibrosis the lesion has to be removed and the two free ends should be sutured together. No traction should be applied to the free ends when suturing in order to avoid future fibrous formation. Approximation of the two ends of the nerve regardless of the direction of fascicles and placing the fascicles alongside each other is called coaptation. Since inferior alveolar nerve is a sensory nerve, often only approximation is sufficient. Sutures are applied to the epineural layer. If neural graft is intended, the most similar nerve to the inferior alveolar nerve in terms of diameter and consistency is the sural nerve and the second most similar is the greater auricular nerve [12,22].

Surgical intervention for a patient suffering from nerve injury has 2 main objectives: resuming the sensory function and managing the pain and discomfort due to nerve injury.

Indications of explorative surgery and nerve reconstruction include:

1. Visible injury

2. Presence of foreign body around the nerve

3. No change in anesthesia or hypoesthesia 2 months after nerve injury

4. Uncontrollable neuropathic pain

Contraindications of explorative surgery and nerve reconstruction include:

1. Signs of improved sensory function based on quantitative sensory testing (QST) which is a method for determining the exact threshold of sensory stimulation with the use of oscillatory, touch, thermal or painful stimuli)

2. Patient admission based on remaining dysfunction or present discomfort

3. Signs of central sensitivity (regional dysesthesia, secondary hyperalgesia)

4. Presence of clinical symptoms with autonomic origin (erythema, swelling, hypersensitivity, burning sensation) which are indicative of autonomic nerve dysfunction rather than sensory nerve injury)

5. Old age, presence of an underlying systemic or neuropathic disease

6. A long time has passed since the injury

7. Patient has unrealistic expectations (demands immediate full recovery or resuming of sensory function with no pain)

8. Neural pains that are not alleviated by local anesthesia [22]

Primary care of a patient with nerve injury includes:

The main goal of primary treatment of nerve injury is to eliminate the progressive cause, and prevent secondary nerve injury to allow formation of a peripheral tissue for maximum recovery of the nerve and avoid secondary neuropathic hypersensitivity. If the injured nerve is exposed, pressure from the foreign body, bony and dental chips, toxic materials or implant if present should be eliminated. The exposed nerve should be washed with isotonic solution and sutured with temporary epineural sutures. Infection and inflammation should be controlled precisely both locally and systemically. Anti-inflammatory medications, opioid analgesics and sedatives should be extensively used in order to control anxiety and minimal stimulation of the CNS. An appropriate method for this purpose is administration of a long acting local block anesthesia. A course of systemic corticosteroids like dexamethasone 8 to 12 mg/day can decrease the perineural inflammation in the first week following surgery [44]. Fast acting anticonvulsants like clonazepam in divided doses of 2 to 10 mg/day can further protect the CNS [45]. Topical lidocaine in the form of gel or 5% patch which is released and absorbed subcutaneously within 12 hours can also be used [46]. Basic examinations should be performed using QST and the injured nerve should be under follow up. The patient should be informed about the nature of nerve injury, importance of tests and examinations, constant and immediate care, possibility of requiring secondary consultation and microscopic reconstructive surgery and possibility of prolonged recovery.

Nerve surgery is categorized into 3 types based on the time of surgery following nerve injury:

1. Primary and immediate surgery: within the first few hours following injury.

2. Delayed surgery: within 14 to 21 days after injury.

3. Secondary surgery: 3 weeks after injury.

Primary surgery is indicated when the nerve is exposed and becomes injured. It is usually performed in cases of trauma, orthognathic surgery, implant surgery, dentoalveolar pathologies and some cases of 3rd molar surgeries. From the biologic point of view, immediate primary surgery is preferred over other types. Despite limitations, primary repair is feasible even in the office. Use of surgical loop is recommended.

Delayed surgery following primary surgery, may also be require which is performed a few weeks following injury when the acute post-op condition of the area has subsided and the site is ready for the definite operation of nerve exposure and microscopic surgery.

Secondary surgery is done for invisible trigeminal nerve injury; this injury is not an uncommon event and requires secondary reconstructive surgery under controlled conditions following informing the patient about the indication of surgery, and explaining the situation according to clinical conditions and repeated QSTs. There is controversy regarding the optimal time for conduction of secondary surgery among researchers [47]. There are 3 reasons why the earlier reconstructive surgery within the first week following injury is preferred:

1. The high capacity for maximum recovery within the first week after surgery

2. Quick intervention can prevent traumatic neuroma from extension and subsequent chronic neuropathic hypersensitivity or fibrosis

3. Technical simplicity of the reconstruction (after a long delay, microscopic surgery would be very difficult due to the contraction and progressive atrophy of the nerve segments, increased collagen precipitation inside and outside the nerve and scarring of Schwann cells)

The first phase of nerve reconstruction includes:

1. Decompression of the injured nerve by extracting the foreign bodies and releasing the scar tissues and other tissues compressed around the nerve.

2. Detection of the injured area, incision and transection of the traumatic neuroma

3. Repair with microscopic sutures through neurorrhaphy (repeated direct anastomosis)

4. Reconstruction through an interstitial graft if neurorrhaphy is not feasible due to the extensive loss of nerve tissue.

Nerve graft: In some cases of severe injury, reconstruction through direct neurorrhaphy is not feasible. Clinical experience shows that distances wider than 15 to 20 mm cannot be repaired through neurorrhaphy and suturing without tension. In such cases, nerve grafting is indicated.

Autogenous graft: Our first choices for a nerve graft are the sural nerve, great auricular nerve, and anti-brachial skin nerve. All these donor nerves are easily accessible and provide sufficient length of the tissue (more than 6 cm)[48-50].In order to avoid tissue fragility, minimum number of sutures should be used. It would be ideal if the nerve is wrapped in a protective biodegradable barrier. The main complications in autogenous grafts are development of a sense of numbness and anesthesia/dysesthesia, and formation of a neuroma at the donor site. In cases where sural nerve is used, there is a risk of defect and difficulty along with hyperesthesia at the lateral and posterior surface of the foot where is in contact with shoes and in the ankle. When the greater auricular nerve is used the patient may experience paresthesia at the lateral side of the neck and at the angle of mandible. This is especially troublesome in patients who have trigeminal neuropathy adjacent to this location. Another problem related to greater auricular nerve is the various diameters of this nerve [51].The greatest technical problem in autogenous nerve graft is the incompatibility in shape, size and number of fascicles between the grafted nerve and the inferior alveolar nerve. The inferior alveolar nerve has an average 2.4 mm diameter and is cylindrical. In comparison, the sural nerve has approximately 2.1 mm diameter versus 1.5 mm diameter of great auricular nerve. Both of these nerves have a significantly smaller number of fascicles than the inferior alveolar nerve [52]. It is not feasible to completely match the fascicles at the time of nerve grafting which amplifies the disorganized regeneration of the axon in between the grafted area [53].

Alternative strategies for autogenous grafts:

An alternative strategy for nerve graft is to use skeletal muscles [54]. To date, there is no definite report regarding the level of sensory recovery of the inferior alveolar nerve. Also, use of arteries and veins has been reported with varying levels of success clinically [55]. Use of vasculature for grafting has been considered because of the minimum tissue invasion and ease of access. However, this method has not shown acceptable results thus far. At present, some have suggested using alloplastic grafts which have caught great attention for their availability and avoiding the morbidity of the donor site. Their biocompatibility and efficacy are for the short grafts only. However, acceptable results have not been reported in this regard either.

Management of sensory function after nerve transposition surgery:

Inferior alveolar nerve transposition for implant placement almost in 100% of cases results in sensory impairment immediately after surgery [10,31,32]. Sensory disturbances are resolved in 84% of cases and in only 16% of patients may this complication be permanent and irreversible [10,24,32,33]. The important issue in management of nerve injury is to inform and educate the patient in this respect. The patient should be educated before and after the surgery and should be well aware that nerve reconstruction may take a long time and he/she may experience paresthesia or dysesthesia for a long period of time. The patient may be taught to massage the area (with lanolin or a moisture absorbing ointment). Massage should be started with mild movements and then the intensity is increased to improve the sense of touch. Massaging is indicated 4 to 6 times a day for 10 to 15 minutes. The first sense that resumes is the sense of cold followed by pain. At this time the patient still has paresthesia in the area. After 4 to 5 months, the patient would be able to differentiate between cold and heat sensations and feels the sharpness of needle with 25 to 30 g pressure. After 6 months, touch, pain and thermal sensations will resume more efficiently [12]. All patients should undergo treatment with low level laser for 10 sessions (4 times a week). The sessions start from the day of surgery. The sensitive area is detected using a simple anesthesia needle and is controlled monthly. The percentage of recovery is calculated by the proportion of the primary area suffering from paresthesia to the final area after 6 months. Researches indicate that chance of spontaneous recovery of the nerve is smaller in women compared to men

[10]. As mentioned earlier, most surgeons believe that sensory disturbances should be considered as a normal predictable state following nerve transposition surgery and not a complication or sequel of treatment [10,32].

Author details

Ali Hassani[1], Mohammad Hosein Kalantar Motamedi[2] and Sarang Saadat[3]

1 Oral and Maxillofacial Surgery, Azad University of Medical Sciences, Tehran, Iran

2 Oral and Maxillofacial Surgery, Trauma Research Center, Baqiyatallah University of Medical Sciences, Tehran, Iran

3 Craniomaxillofacial Research Center, Tehran University of Medical Sciences, Tehran, Iran

References

[1] J.M. Hirsch, P.I. Branemark. Fixture stability and nerve function after transposition and lateralization of the inferior alveolar nerve and fixture installation. Br J Oral Maxillofac Surg.1995;33(5):276-281.

[2] Thoma Kh, Holland DJ. Atrophy of the mandible.Oral Surg Oral Med Oral Pathol. 1951;4(12):1477-95.

[3] Rocchietta I, Fontana F, Simion M. Clinical outcomes of vertical bone augmentation to enable dental implant placement: a systematic review.Clin Periodontol. 2008;35:203-15.

[4] Boyne PJ, Cooksey DE. Use of cartilage and bone implants in restoration of edentulous ridges.J Am Dent Assoc. 1965;71(6):1426-35.

[5] Chang CS, Matukas VJ, Lemons JE.Histologic study of hydroxylapatite as an implant material for mandibular augmentation.J Oral Maxillofac Surg. 1983;41(11):729-37.

[6] Jensen OT. Combined hydroxylapatite augmentation and lip-switch vestibuloplasty in the mandible..Oral Surg Oral Med Oral Pathol. 1985;60(4):349-55.

[7] Egbert M, Stoelinga PJ, Blijdorp PA, de Koomen HA. The "three-piece" osteotomy and interpositional bone graft for augmentation of the atrophic mandible.J Oral Maxillofac Surg. 1986;44(9):680-7.

[8] Matras H. A review of surgical procedures designed to increase the functional height of the resorbed alveolar ridge.Int Dent J. 1983;33(4):332-8.

[9] Vasconcelos Jde A, Avila GB, Ribeiro JC, Dias SC, Pereira LJ. Inferior alveolar nerve transposition with involvement of the mental foramen for implant placement.Med Oral Patol Oral Cir Bucal.2008;13(11):E722-5.

[10] Jensen O, Nock D.Inferior alveolar nerve repositioning in conjunction with placement of osseointegrated implants: a case report.Oral Surg Oral Med Oral Pathol. 1987;63(3):263-8.

[11] Rosenquist B.Fixture placement posterior to the mental foramen with transpositioning of the inferior alveolar nerve.Int J Oral Maxillofac Implants. 1992;7(1):45-50.

[12] Yaghmaei M.Mandibular Canal (clinical Aspects).1st ed.Tehran: Karvar Publishers; 2010.

[13] Hu KS, Yun HS, Hur MS, Kwon HJ, Abe S, Kim HJ. Branching patterns and intraosseous course of the mental nerve. J Oral Maxillofac Surg. 2007;65(11):2288-94.

[14] Sanchis JM, Peñarrocha M, Soler F.Bifid mandibular canal. J Oral Maxillofac Surg. 2003;61(4):422-4.

[15] Stella JP, Tharanon W.A precise radiographic method to determine the location of the inferior alveolar canal in the posterior edentulous mandible: implications for dental implants. Part2: Technique.Int J Oral Maxillofac Implants. 1990;5(1):23-9.

[16] Stella JP, Tharanon W.A precise radiographic method to determine the location of the inferior alveolar canal in the posterior edentulous mandible: implications for dental implants. Part 1: Technique.Int J Oral Maxillofac Implants. 1990;5(1):15-22

[17] Kieser J. Kieser D. Hauman T.The Course and Distribution of the Inferior Alveolar Nerve in the Edentulous Mandible. J Cranio fac Surg..2005;16(1):6-9.

[18] Chrcanovic BR, Custodio AL. Inferior alveolar nerve lateral transposition. Oral Maxillofac Surg. 2009;13(4):213-9.

[19] Wadu SG, Penhall B, Townsend GC.Morphological variability of the human inferior alveolar nerve. Clin Anat. 1997;10(2):82-7.

[20] Choukas NC, Toto PD, Nolan RF.A histologic study of the regeneration of the inferior alveolar nerve.J Oral Surg. 1974;32(5):347-52.

[21] Yaghmaei M, Mashhadiabbas F, Shahabi S, Zafarbakhsh A, Yaghmaei S, Khojasteh A. Histologic evaluation of inferior alveolar lymphatics: an anatomic study. Oral Surg Oral Med Oral Pathol Oral Radiol Endod. 2011 Feb 16.

[22] Van Geffen GJ, Moayeri N, Bruhn J, Scheffer GJ, Chan VW, Groen GJ.Correlation between ultrasound imaging, cross-sectional anatomy, and histology of the brachial plexus: a review. Reg Anesth Pain Med. 2009;34(5):490-7.

[23] Hupp J.R. Ellis E.Tucker M.R.Contemporary Oral and Maxillofacial surgery.5th ed.Missouri:Mosby Elsevier;2008.p.281,285,620-622.

[24] Seddon HJ.A Classification of Nerve Injuries. Br Med J. 1942 Aug 29;2(4260):237-9.

[25] Sunderland S.A classification of peripheral nerve injuries producing loss of function. Brain.1951;74(4):491-516.

[26] Poort LJ, van Neck JW, van der Wal KG. Sensory testing of inferior alveolar nerve injuries: a review of methods used in prospective studies.J Oral Maxillofac Surg. 2009;67(2):292-300.

[27] Kahnberg KE, Ridell A. Transposition of the mental nerve in orthognathic surgery. J Oral Maxillofac Surg. 1987;45(4):315-8.

[28] Lindh C, Petersson A.Radiologic examination for location of the mandibular canal: a comparison between panoramic radiography and conventional tomography.Int J Oral Maxillofac Implants.1989;4(3):249-53.

[29] Babbush CA,Hahn JA,Krauser JT,Rosenlicht JL.Dental Implants:The Art and Science, 2th Ed. London:Saunders Elsevier ; 2010,232-250.

[30] Rosenquist Bo.Implant Placement in Combination With Nerve Transpositioning: Experiences With the First 100 Cases.Int J Oral Maxillofac Implants.1994: 9(5):522-531.

[31] Rosenquist BE.Nerve transpositioning to facilitate implant placement. Dent Econ. 1995;85(10):92-3.

[32] Kan JY, Lozada JL, Goodacre CJ, Davis WH, Hanisch O. Endosseous implant placement in conjunction with inferior alveolar nerve transposition: an evaluation of neurosensory disturbance.Int J Oral Maxillofac Implants. 1997;12(4):463-71.

[33] Peleg M, Mazor Z, Chaushu G, Garg AK. Lateralization of the inferior alveolar nerve with simultaneous implant placement: a modified technique.Int J Oral Maxillofac Implants2002;17(1):101-6.

[34] Friberg B, Ivanoff CJ, Lekholm U. Inferior alveolar nerve transposition in combination with Branemark implant treatment. Int J Periodontics Restorative Dent. 1992;12(6):440-9.

[35] Hashemi HM.Neurosensory function following mandibular nerve lateralization for placement of implants.Int J Oral Maxillofac Surg. 2010;39(5):452-6.

[36] Smiler DG. Repositioning the inferior alveolar nerve for placement of endosseous implants: technical note.Int J Oral Maxillofac Implants. 1993;8(2):145-50.

[37] Yoshimoto M, Konig B Jr, Allegrini S Jr, de Carvalho Lopes C, Carbonari MJ, Liberti EA, Adami N Jr. Bone healing after the inferior alveolar nerve lateralization: a histologic study in rabbits (Oryctolagus cuniculus).J Oral Maxillofac Surg. 2004;62:131-5.

[38] Kahnberg KE, Henry PJ, Tan AE, Johansson CB, Albrektsson T.Tissue regeneration adjacent to titanium implants placed with simultaneous transposition of the inferior dental nerve: a study in dogs. Int J Oral Maxillofac Implants. 2000;15(1):119-24.

[39] Brasileiro BF, Van Sickels JE.A modified sagittal split ramus osteotomy for hemimandibular hyperplasia and simultaneous inferior alveolar nerve repositioning. J Oral Maxillofac Surg. 2011 Dec;69(12):e533-41

[40] Kraut RA, Chahal O. Management of patients with trigeminal nerve injuries after mandibular implant placement. J Am Dent Assoc. 2002;133(10):1351-4.

[41] Kubilius R. Sabalys G. Juodzbalys G.Gedrimas V.Traumatic Damage to the Inferior Alveolar Nerve Sustained in Course of Dental Implantation.Possibility of Prevention.Stomatologija,Baltic Dent Maxillofac.2004; 6:106-10.

[42] Khullar SM, Brodin P, Barkvoll P, et al: Preliminary study of low-level laser for treatment of long-standing sensory aberrations in the inferior alveolar nerve. J Oral Maxillofac Surg 54:2, 1996

[43] Matsen FA,Winquist RA,Krugmire RB. Diagnosis and management of compartment syndromes. J bone joint surg Am.1980;62(2):286-291.

[44] Seo K et al..Efficacy of steroid treatment for sensory impairment after orthognathic surgery. Oral Maxillofac surg 2004; 62:1193.

[45] Bartusch SL. Et al..Clonazepam for the treatment of lancinating phantom pain. Clin J Pain 1996;12:59.

[46] Rowbotham MC et al.Lidocaine patch: double-blind controlled study of a new treatment method for postherpetic neuralgia.J Pain.1996;65: 39.

[47] Davis H, Ohrnell LO, Larson C, et al. Lateralizing of the inferior alveolar nerve to allow fixture placement. Proceedings of the UCLA Symposium on Implants in the Partially Edentulous Patient. Los Angeles, 1990:28–31.

[48] Susarla SM et al..Dose early repair of lingual nerve injuries improve functional sensory recovery?. J oral maxillofac surg;2007:65:1070.

[49] Brammer JP, Epker BN. Anatomic-histologic survey of the sural nerve: implications for inferior alveolar nerve grafting.J Oral Maxillofac Surg. 1988;46(2):111-7.

[50] Eppley BL, Snyders RV Jr. Microanatomic analysis of the trigeminal nerve and potential nerve graft donor sites.J Oral Maxillofac Surg. 1991;49(6):612-8.

[51] McCormick SU, Buchbinder D, McCormick SA, Stark M. Microanatomic analysis of the medial antebrachial nerve as a potential donor nerve in maxillofacial grafting.J Oral Maxillofac Surg. 1994;52(10):1022-5.

[52] Takasaki Y, Noma H, Kitami T, Shibahara T, Sasaki K. Reconstruction of the inferior alveolar nerve by autologous graft: a retrospective study of 20 cases examining donor nerve length.Bull Tokyo Dent Coll. 2003;44(2):29-35.

[53] Pogrel MA, Renaut A, Schmidt B, Ammar A. The relationship of the lingual nerve to the mandibular third molar region: an anatomic study.J Oral Maxillofac Surg. 1995;53(10):1178-81.

[54] Rath EM. Skeletal muscle autograft for repair of the human inferior alveolar nerve: a case report.J Oral Maxillofac Surg. 2002;60(3):330-4

[55] Pogrel MA, Maghen A. The use of autogenous vein grafts for inferior alveolar and lingual nerve reconstruction.J Oral Maxillofac Surg. 2001;59(9):985-8.

[56] Miloro M, Stoner JA. Subjective outcomes following sural nerve harvest. Oral Maxillofac Surg. 2005;63(8):1150-4.

Orthognathic Surgery of Maxillofacial Deformities

Rigid Fixation of Intraoral Vertico-Sagittal Ramus Osteotomy for Mandibular Prognathism

Kazuma Fujimura and Kazuhisa Bessho

Additional information is available at the end of the chapter

1. Introduction

The standard surgical treatment for mandibular prognathism is sagittal split ramus osteotomy (SSRO) if the proximal and distal segments of the ramus require fixing with screws or metal plates. In this procedure, however, it is frequently difficult to avoid neurosensory disturbance (NSD) of the inferior alveolar nerve (IAN) when the posterior margin of the ramus curves inward or when the ramus is thin (Fig 1A,B).

This report describes a new alternative procedure, intraoral vertico-sagittal ramus osteotomy (IVSRO) reported by Choung in 1992. [1] It is a modification of SSRO and intraoral vertical ramus osteotomy (IVRO). It is supposed that IVSRO is more suitable for, mandibles with a 'V' shape seen in adult Asians as compared to mandibles of Caucasians who have 'U' shaped mandibles. One of the main advantages of IVSRO is that it avoids IAN damage, because the ramus can be split parallel to the original sagittal plane posterior to the point between the mandibular canal and the lateral cortical bone plate immediately in front of the antilingular prominence. In this method the anterior border of the proximal segment is partially removed at the beginning of the osteotomy procedure as described by Kitajima et al. in 1989. [2] Another advantage of IVSRO is that the area in which screws can be inserted is relatively large; the subcoronoid area on the distal segment and subcondylar area on the proximal segment are engaged. These segments can be fixed in these areas with bicortical bone screws, without a cheek incision (Fig 1AC). This chapter introduces this procedure and the technique of rigid fixation of IVSRO for treatment of mandibular prognathism.

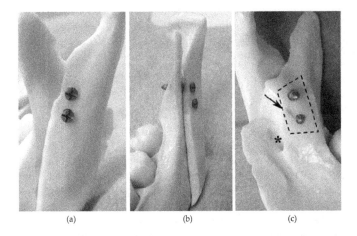

(a)   (b)   (c)

Figure 1. (a) Rigid fixation of intraoral vertico-sagittal ramus osteotomy using a mandibular model. Left mandibular ramus lateral view showing bone overlap and bicortical screw engagement. Screws can be inserted into the subcoronoid area on the distal segment in the subcondylar area on the proximal segment; (b) Left mandibular ramus frontal view showing bicortical engagement of screws; (c) Left mandibular ramus medial view showing relatively large area for screw insertion (*dashed rectangular area*). *Arrow* indicates lingula of mandible. *Asterisk* indicates mandibular foramen.

2. Technique

Osteotomy of the ramus via IVSRO is a modified version of the 'straight IVSRO'. [1] Briefly, the lateral aspect of the ramus is exposed from the sigmoid notch to the antegonial notch. To avoid damaging the IAN and the maxillary artery, the medial aspect of the ramus may also be exposed carefully from the sigmoid notch area to the lingula and the posterior border of the ramus, as in SSRO. [3] To avoid a fracture or bad split, the full thickness of the sigmoid notch is cut with a fissure bur, reciprocating saw, oscillating saw or ultrasonic surgical device inferiorly along the planned decortication line until the bone marrow is exposed. This process, full-thickness cutting of the sigmoid notch, is the most important and most technically difficult step of the IVSRO procedure. A wedge-shaped decortication of the lateral aspect of the ramus from the sigmoid notch to the antegonial notch is performed using a flat-top, cylindrical fissure bur parallel to the original sagittal plane until the bone marrow is exposed. [4] A bone spatula and an osteotome are used for vertical osteotomy along almost the entire sagittal plane to the medial posterior border of the ramus. The distal segment is then repositioned posteriorly, and intermaxillary fixation (IMF) is performed. The inner aspect of the decorticated distal segment is spontaneously overlapped on the proximal segment. The subcoronoid area and the subcondylar area in each segment also overlap. These segments can be fixed using bicortical bone screws. A 90° screw driver system (eg, angled drilling system and insertion screws with a 12mm screw length) is used with an intraorally (Fig 1 A–C).

When the two segments are fixed rigidly, IMF is usually not required after surgery. However, a favorable outcome is usually obtained with IMF for about 3 days to prevent postoperative bleeding and to aid in wound healing. To stabilize the occlusion postoperatively, intermaxillary elastics are applied for about 2-3 months after release of IMF.

3. Discussion

The main advantage of rigid fixation IVSRO over SSRO in treating prognathism, when the posterior margin of the ramus curves inward or the ramus is thin, may be the decreased risk of postoperative NSD. The incidence of long-term NSD of the lower lip and chin in IVSRO is 0% to 6% [1,5,6] compared with 39% to 85% [7-11] for SSRO. Although the osteotomy plane is between the mandibular canal and the lateral cortical plate of the ramus as in SSRO, damage to the IAN can be avoided because the osteotomy is performed from a point in front of the foramen between the mandibular canal and the immediately medial lateral cortical bone.[1, 2] making it possible to strip the lateral cortical bone from the bone marrow. Although a low incidence of NSD is also observed with IVRO, [10,12] rigid fixation with screws or bone plates has several disadvantages, including technical difficulty [10,13] and rotation of the condyle to the laterally.[1] IVSRO is distinguished by flat and larger contact areas of segments and more favorable healing of the medulla to the cortex than the cortex-to-cortex healing of IVRO. [1] In SSRO, the excess overlap of the anterior edge of the proximal segment must be removed to fit the two segments and/or prevent distal rotation of the proximal segment. [14] In IVSRO, there is no excess overlap of the proximal segment. It is easy to check the position of the distal segment after osteotomy because the anterior area of the proximal segment is removed beforehand; hence, the subcoronoid area of the distal segment and the subcondylar area of the proximal segment can be used for insertion of screws. The area available for screw insertion is relatively large and the ends of the inserted screws may be viewed at the medial aspect of the distal segment because, at the internal oblique ridge, the bone thickness of this subcoronoid area in the distal segment is relatively thin compared with the retromolar areas as in SSRO. Therefore, in many patients, a 90° angle screwdriver system with 12-mm length screws can be used without drilling through a trocar inserted through the skin (Fig 2 A–C).

4. Conclusion

When planning rigid fixation using IVSRO, the following conditions are preferable: Mandibular setback (about ≥ 5 mm) and counterclockwise rotation. Because this osteotomy procedure has a large contact area between the proximal and distal segments, compared with IVRO, the segments are usually fixed with screws in only the setback side for horizontal rotation for mandibular asymmetry (Fig 2C). Additional studies including the development of osteotomy instruments and drilling systems to simplify the surgical procedure of IVSRO are needed to validate the advantages of this procedure.

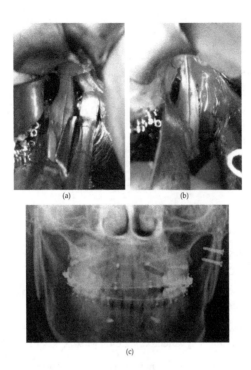

Figure 2. (a) Intraoral vertico-sagittal ramus osteotomy of the left ramus (frontal view). A 90° angled screwdriver drilling system and insertion screws, 12-mm in length; (b) Two 12-mm screws 2.4 mm in diameter inserted intraorally.

Author details

Kazuma Fujimura and Kazuhisa Bessho

*Address all correspondence to: fujimura@kuhp.kyotou.ac.jp

Department of Oral and Maxillofacial Surgery, Graduate School of Medicine, Kyoto University, Kyoto, Japan

References

[1] Choung PH: A new osteotomy for the correction of mandibular prognathism: Techniques and rationale of the intraoral verticosagittal ramus osteotomy. J Craniomaxillofac Surg 20:153, 1992

[2] Kitajima T, Handa Y, Naitoh K: A modification of the sagittal splitting technique ensuring that the osteotomy split lies immediately medial to the lateral cortex. J Craniomaxillofac Surg 17:53, 1989

[3] Fujimura K, Segami N, Kobayashi S: Anatomical study of the complications of intraoral vertico-sagittal ramus osteotomy. J Oral Maxillofac Surg 64:384, 2006

[4] Fujimura K, Segami N, Sato J, et al: Advantages of intraoral verticosagittal ramus osteotomy in skeletofacial deformity patients with temporomandibular joint disorders. J Oral Maxillofac Surg 62:1246, 2004

[5] Lima Júnior SM, Granato R, Marin C, et al: Analysis of 40 cases of intraoral verticosagittal ramus osteotomies to treat dentofacial deformities. J Oral Maxillofac Surg 67:1840, 2009

[6] Hashemi HM: Evaluation of intraoral verticosagittal ramus osteotomy for correction of mandibular prognathism: A 10-year study. J Oral Maxillofac Surg 66:509, 2008

[7] Walter JM Jr, Gregg JM: Analysis of postsurgical neurologic alteration in the trigeminal nerve. J Oral Surg 37:410, 1979

[8] MacIntosh RB: Experience with the sagittal osteotomy of the mandibular ramus: A 13-year review. J Maxillofac Surg 9:151, 1981

[9] Nishioka GJ, Zysset MK, Van Sickels JE: Neurosensory disturbance with rigid fixation of the bilateral sagittal split osteotomy. J Oral Maxillofac Surg 45:20, 1987

[10] Hall HD: Mandibular prognathism, in Bell WH (ed): Modern Practice in Orthognathic and Reconstructive Surgery. Philadelphia, PA, WB Saunders, 1992, p 2111

[11] Westermark A, Bystedt H, von Konow L: Inferior alveolar nerve function after mandibular osteotomies. Br J Oral Maxillofac Surg 36:425, 1998

[12] van Merkesteyn JP, Groot RH, Van Leeuwaarden R, et al: Intra-operative complications in sagittal and vertical ramus osteotomies. Int J Oral Maxillofac Surg 16:665, 1987

[13] Ghali GE, Sikes JW Jr: Intraoral vertical ramus osteotomy as the preferred treatment for mandibular prognathism. J Oral Maxillofac Surg 58:313, 2000

[14] Sickels JEV, Jeter TS, Aragon SB: Orthognathic surgery, in Bell WH (ed): Modern Practice in Orthognathic and Reconstructive Surgery. Philadelphia, PA, WB Saunders, 1992, p 1980

Chapter 5

Basic and Advanced Operative Techniques in Orthognathic Surgery

F. Arcuri, M. Giarda, L. Stellin, A. Gatti, M. Nicolotti, M. Brucoli, A. Benech and P. Boffano

Additional information is available at the end of the chapter

1. Introduction

Orthognathic surgical procedures have been developed to reposition the jaws and have been traditionally used in the dentate patient to correct a skeletal malocclusion; these procedures are usually carried out with orthodontic control of the dentition to produce the best results. The majority of the clinical cases of maxillary deformities can be solved by three basic osteotomies: the LeFort I type maxillary osteotomy (LFI), the bilateral sagittal split osteotomy of the mandible (BSSO) and the horizontal sliding osteotomy of the mandibular symphysis (genioplasty).The LeFort I osteotomy, as described by Obwegeser in 1965, manages the midface; it can be performed as a single-piece monobloc technique or it can be executed as a multisegment procedure or with a distraction approach such as SARPE (Surgically Assisted Rapid Palatal Expansion). The BSSO and the genioplasty, described by the same author in 1955 and in 1957, respectively, allows the surgeon to modify the mandible.[1-3]

Orthognathic surgery can require the execution of codified subapical osteotomies to manage peculiar dento-alveolar discrepancies such as: the segmental anterior maxillary osteotomy according to Wassmund, the segmental posterior maxillary osteotomy according to Schuchardt and the segmental anterior mandibular osteotomy according to Köle.[4-6]Moreover, there are osteotomy well described in the scientific literature but now rarely used in the common practice such as: the intraoral vertical subcondylar osteotomy (Hebert, 1970), the median mandibular osteotomy, the maxillary-zygomatic osteotomy and the quadrangular Le Fort I osteotomy.[7-9]Historically, orthognathic surgery is used to correct dento-facial malocclusion and it is a common practice in maxillo-facial surgery; however, based on an extensive review associated with our experience, we report peculiar clinical scenarios, different from simple malocclusion, where orthognathic surgery is a precious tool.

2. Obstructive sleep apnea syndrome

Continuous positive airway pressure therapy (CPAP) is the first line treatment for patients affected by Obstructive Sleep Apnea Syndrome (OSAS). CPAP prevents upper airway collapse, relieves symptoms such daytime sleepiness and decreases the cardiovascular accidents events. However, this treatment has poor patient compliance. An alternative approach to CPAP is upper airway surgery. The goal of surgery is to increase the posterior airway space and decrease the resistance to airflow, removing the site or sites of upper airway collapse.

Different surgical approaches have been proposed in the literature: tracheostomy, uvulopalatopharyngoplasty, hyoid suspension, partial glossectomy, lingual suspension, tongue base resection, genioglossus advancement and maxillomandibular advancement (MMA). Scientific literature considers MMA as the most effective surgical treatment for the management of adult OSAS. Surgical success and long-term stability confirms the efficacy and safety of this procedure. Tracheostomy is the surgical treatment for OSA patients with a success of 100% because it bypasses the site of collapse; however, it is indicated as a treatment of last resort after the failure of other surgical procedures. The reported surgical success rate for soft tissue surgical procedures is approximately 40-60%. MMA enlarges the pharyngeal space by expanding the skeletal framework; MMA is currently the most effective surgical treatment for the management of OSAS in adults.

To assess the surgical success and the long term stability both objective and subjective parameters are generally considered before surgery (T0), at 6 months after surgery (T1) and at follow up (T2). Objective examinations are commonly evaluated by upper airway fibroscopy during the Mueller's manoeuvre, by lateral cephalometry and by polysomnography. Subjective examinations can be evaluated by Epwhorth Sleepiness Scale (ESS) questionnaire.

With upper airway endoscopic evaluation performed by flexible fiberoptic endoscope in supine position during the Mueller's manoeuvre, it can be assessed:

1. the localization of collapse (N: Nose, O: Oropharynx, H: Hypopharynx);

2. the pattern of collapse (c: Circular, t: Transversal, AP: Antero-Posterior);

3. the grade of collapse (grade 0, 1, 2, 3, 4) (NOH classification).[10-12]

With lateral cephalometry, performed on latero-lateral teleradiography by the same operator, it is possible to evaluate the sskeletal relationship by angular measurements (SNA, SNB) and the posterior air space (PAS) between the base of the tongue and the posterior wall of the pharynx. With polysomnography it can be possible to evaluate the average number of apneas and hypopneas per hour during sleep (AHI), the average number of oxyhemoglobin desaturation per hour during sleep (ODI) and the average time spent with oxyhemoglobin saturation below 90% during sleep ($SaO_2 < 90$).

Results of OSA surgical treatment are divided into "surgical success" and "surgical cure". Surgical success is defined as an AHI < 20 events/hour. Surgical cure is defined as an AHI < 5 events/hour after surgical procedure. Holty and Guilleminault performed a meta-analysis regarding the clinical efficacy of MMA in treating OSAS. Six hundred twenty- seven adults with OSAS underwent to MMA. The mean AHI decreased from 63.9 events/h to 9.5 events/h following surgery. The surgical success and cure rates were 86 ± 30.9% and 43.2 ± 11.7% respectively. Also they observed the maintenance of surgical success rate at 44 months after surgery.[13, 14]

The analysis of skeletal cephalometric values (SNA and SNB) at T1 and at T2 does not show generally significant differences, confirming the long-term stability of skeletal advancement. According to the literature, the postoperative PAS (T1) has commonly an increase. At T2 the PAS maintains stable values. The skeletal advancement is commonly 1 cm for each jaw. Lye et al. found a statistically significant correlation between the degree of maxillary advancement and reduction in AHI. However, others have reported no association between the degree of maxillary advancement and improvement in AHI after MMA. MMA is generally safe with a reported major surgical complication maxillary (ischemic necrosis, cardiac complication) rate of 1%, minor complication (mandibular relapse, facial paresthesia, temporomandibular joint disorder) rate of 3.1% and no reported deaths.

OSAS is a chronic disease, so the treatment goal is the control of the symptoms and the control of OSAS-related risks by reducing the severity of the disorder. Surgical success and long term stability of outcomes confirm the efficacy and safety of MMA for treatment of OSAS. However a continuous follow up of these patients is necessary to control their lifestyle and to detect any possible relapse.[15] (Fig. 1 a-d)

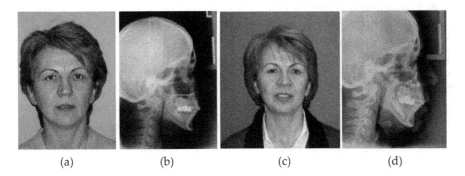

(a)   (b)   (c)   (d)

Figure 1. a) Preoperative frontal view. b) Preoperative radiographic examination. c) Photograph after bimaxillary surgery for advancement. d) Postoperative radiograph demonstrating successful advancement.

3. Preprosthetic technique in orthognathic surgery

Orthognathic surgery can be performed on the edentulous patient to correct discrepancies between the jaws, followed by the placement of implants to rehabilitate the maxillary bones; different surgical approaches and technical variations have been proposed.

This reconstructive method has the advantages over other commonly used preprosthetic techniques of simultaneously allowing the placement of osseointegrated implants, while correcting an unfavourable intermaxillary relationship and improving facial esthetics. [16-18]

Since the 1970s osseointegrated implants have played an important role in oral and maxillofacial reconstruction. Although the success of this method for edentulous jaws with sufficient bone height, patients with an atrophic maxilla and mandible continue to be difficult cases for an optimal outcome in terms of esthetics and function. This condition is characterized by the lack of bone for implants and a reverse maxillomandibular relationship; the progressive loss of alveolar bone height leads to less volume available for the implants with a high rate of surgical failure. Vertically directed resorption increases the interarch space; the projection of the maxilla diminishes in the sagittal plane with change of the intermaxillary relationships and a pseudoprognathism. The combination of loss of projection and diminished vertical bone height results in collapse of the soft tissues of the midface resulting in a more aged face.

Orthognathic surgical procedures have been initially described to reposition the jaws and have been traditionally used in the dentate patient to correct a skeletal malocclusion; these procedures are usually carried out with orthodontic control. Moreover, these procedures are used on the edentulous patient to correct the discrepancies between the maxilla and the mandible associated with the placement of implants to rehabilitate the oral cavity.[19-21] This reconstructive method has the advantages over other commonly used preprosthetic techniques of simultaneously allowing the placement of osseointegrated implants while correcting an unfavourable intermaxillary relationship and reversing facial aging. However, LeFort I osteotomy as a preprosthetic procedure for the atrophic edentulous maxilla is a technically demanding procedure and there are some complications such as infection, hemorrhage, aseptic and avascular necrosis, fractures of the maxilla, bone exposure and oroantral fistulas.

LeFort I osteotomy with interpositional and onlay bone grafts followed by implants' placement is one of the most common methods to manage a deficient vertical and horizontal maxillary dimension. However, this is a two-step procedure involving significant surgery with considerable morbidity at the donor site with a high rate of bone graft resorption. Recently surgeons use a computer-assisted software, which enables them to insert implants after a digital analysis of the residual alveolar and basal bone. This method offers surgeons the possibility of visualizing anatomic structures, evaluating implant position and inclination and to accurately insert implants. Implant-prosthetic rehabilitation can be difficult and affords both functional and psychological improvement. Computer assisted surgery can be the treatment of choice for these conditions; and the insertion of implants in the presence of marked bony defects can be simplified (Fig. 2 a-g).[22, 23]

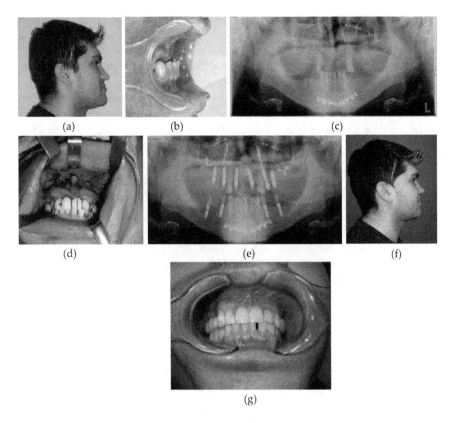

Figure 2. a) Clinical examination demonstrating a prognathic and reverse maxillary relationship. b) Clinical view revealing partial edentulism of the maxillary and mandibular arches with a severe atrophy of the upper jaw. c) Preoperative orthopantomograph showing the osteosynthesis plates after craniofacial trauma. d) Photograph demonstrating a sequence of the LeFort 1 osteotomy. e) Postoperative radiographic examination showing the adequate osteosynthesis after LeFort I osteotomy and dental implants. f) Postoperative lateral view demonstrating an adequate morphology. g) Occlusal view showing an optimal healing of the intraoral tissues.

4. Post-traumatic malocclusion

Facial fractures must be reduced as soon as possible to ensure a proper result; despite a careful surgical technique skeletal and soft-tissue deformities can persist. Orbito-zygomatic, nasal and occlusion problems can occur and result in an unsatisfactory outcome. Orthognathic surgery can be used to manage dentofacial post-traumatic deformities, coordinated with orthodontic and prosthodontic techniques. Management follows the basic rules for correcting primary malocclusion such as: preoperative detailed analysis with clinical records and cephalometric evaluation, well-established orthognathic surgical procedures and postoperative care.

Post-traumatic malocclusion can occur as a result in delayed treatment for unfavourable clinical conditions of the patient such as neurological, abdominal and thoracic injuries; otherwise it can be the squeal of a bad surgical outcome after a primary surgical treatment. Although post-traumatic deformities of the midface are managed with osteotomy in the lines of fracture such as in the malpositioned zygoma, orthognathic surgery, along with preoperative and postoperative orthodontic treatment, reposition the maxilla and the mandible in the preoperative three-dimensional position. Unsatisfactory outcomes of primary management of complex midfacial fractures can result in displacement of the jaws in the three planes of the space, resulting in altered dental and skeletal relationships.

According to the basic rules of orthognathic surgery, LeFort I single or multisegmental osteotomy and bilateral sagittal split osteotomy are indicated, eventually with bone grafts to support the movement of the jaws in the sagittal, vertical, and transverse planes. Treatment planning include endodontics assessment, orthodontic therapy, prosthodontic rehabilitation. Preoperative records such as dental casts, clinical photographs and radiographs, should be obtained to guarantee a satisfactory result. Mandibular or maxillary non-union is commonly managed with debridement of the original fracture with realignment of the occlusion, autologous bone grafting and osteosynthesis with miniplates and screws.

Post-traumatic maxillary deformities after LeFort fractures show midface retrusion, low facial height, anterior open bite, and mandibular overclosure for posterior displacement of the maxilla; moreover anterior cephalic telescoping of the mandible can be found from inferior pull of the pterygoid musculature on the pterygoid plates. LeFort I osteotomy to correct the malocclusion is often the easiest solution, regardless of the primary fracture. Moreover, if occlusal correction is planned, attention to the transverse dentoalveolar relationships should be addressed to determine if maxillary segmental osteotomies are required or preoperative orthodontic therapy is needed.[24]

Conversely, the most common fracture of the mandible which leads to post-traumatic malocclusion is related to the condyle. Discussion about the primary indication for surgery or closed treatment both in children and in adult patients is beyond the scope of this chapter. However, post-traumatic malocclusion with asymmetry caused by unilateral condylar process fractures can be managed with an osteotomy on the affected side or sometimes on both sides. A symmetric anterior open bite caused by bilateral condylar process fractures presents a surgical dilemma. It can be corrected with maxillary and/or mandibular osteotomies, according to dental, skeletal and esthetics issues. Finally, masticatory dysfunction is primarily related to the post-traumatic malocclusion. However, diminished mandibular movement can also lead to oral dysfunction. Trismus may be the result of temporomandibular joint (TMJ) dysfunction. TMJ dysfunction needs to be managed by a variety of techniques such as: occlusal splints, physiotherapy, and surgical procedures of the TMJ.[25] (Fig. 3 a-d)

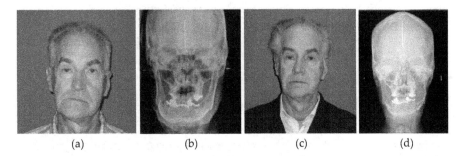

(a)   (b)   (c)   (d)

Figure 3. a) Clinical view of a post-traumatic mandibular laterodeviation. b) Radiographic evaluation. c) Postoperative condition showing facial balance. d) Postoperative control radiograph.

5. Maxillofacial approach

There are peculiar clinical circumstances where orthognathic surgery can solve the problem. Extraction of deeply located impacted inferior wisdom molars in close relationship with the inferior alveolar nerve (IAN)[26] or large cysts can be successfully removed by a bilateral sagittal split osteotomy (BSSO) of the mandible.[27]

Although enucleation and/or curettage together with bone removal is the treatment of choice for deeply located mandibular cysts, BSSO can be considered as a valid alternative to the conventional surgical approaches to achieve an adequate exposure of the region of the angle. In this region, the bone between the nerve and the external cortex is thick; therefore, bone removal by a buccal approach can be troublesome, increasing the risk of nerve injury.

The same discussion can be addressed for deeply located wisdom molars where the standard buccal approach poses an unacceptable risk to damage the IAN with excessive bone removal. However, although BSSO guarantees a wide exposure of the IAN, the dental roots and the cystic wall, it is still associated with complications such as: neurosensory disturbances, nonunion, malocclusion, unfavourable fractures, infections and hemorrhage.

Moreover, the mandibular osteotomy can be used as a decompressive technique in case of endodontic overfilling involving the mandibular canal with a potential risk of permanent IAN's injury.[28] Iatrogenic injury to the IAN after endodontic treatment of the posterior mandibular teeth is a well described complication which may lead to sensory disturbances such as pain, hypoesthesia, paresthesia, and dysesthesia of the chin and the lower lip. Two mechanisms are involved in the damage of the nerve: the chemical neurotoxicity of the components of the endodontic material and the mechanical pressure of the material injected into the mandibular canal.

Although decortication in association to apicectomy is considered the treatment of choice for removing endodontic paste, BSSO is also an adequate alternative. In the region of the mandibular angle, the bone is thick and the view is poor; then, decortication with apicectomy removes bone, while increasing the risk of nerve injury with a "blind" approach. However, as the degree of nerve injury increases with time, early surgical decompression of the IAN must be performed, regardless of the surgical approach.

LeFort I osteotomy and its variations are extensively used to approach nasal, paranasal and skull base regions. The removal of cranio-cervical lesions from the sphenoid to the fourth cervical vertebra between the carotids can be relatively easy with the transmaxillary approach.

Lesions that are intrasellar (pituitary tumors, craniopharyngiomas, Rathke's cysts) are frequently approached endoscopically. However, when an extensive exposure is needed, the transmaxillary approach gives a wider access to the clival lesions with superior and inferior extension for both benign neoplasms (angiofibroma, chordoma, fibrous dysplasia meningocele, aneurysm) and malignant tumours (malignant acinic cell, adenocarcinoma, adenoid cystic carcinoma, chondrosarcoma, olfactory neuroblastoma, sarcoma).Complications related to the transmaxillary approach include: injury of the infraorbital nerve, dental roots, tooth buds and lacrimal duct. Moreover avascular and aseptic necrosis of the soft-tissue, bone, and teeth, along with malocclusion, oronasal fistula and velopharyngeal dysfunction are well described.[29]

6. Clefts and craniofacial syndromes

Craniofacial morphology of patients affected by lip and palate cleft is characterized by a retrusion of the maxilla. The maxilla shows a various degree of skeletal, soft tissue, and dental deficiency. Maxilla shows clockwise rotation, with an increase of the anterior height of the mandible and a decrease in the posterior height of the maxilla. The severity of the malocclusion and the facial asymmetry indicates the surgical and orthodontic therapy. Surgical procedures performed during childhood are lip and palate clefts reconstruction, alveolar cleft repair and pharyngeal flap. Mild discrepancies of the jaws may be camouflaged by the orthodontic therapy during childhood; however, at the end of the skeletal growth, orthognathic surgery can be the treatment of choice for some cases.[30, 31]

Orthognathic surgery can be performed for the correction of malocclusion in patients with craniofacial syndromes (Crouzon, Apert, Treacher Collins, Hemifacial microsomia, Goldenhar syndrome). Treacher Collins syndrome is characterized by agenesis of the zygomatic bone and hypoplasia of the greater wings of the sphenoid. The zygomatic arch can be absent or hypoplastic; the maxilla and the mandible show a various degree of hypoplasia. Early correction of mandibular defects can be performed with distractors; however, bilateral sagittal split osteotomy (BSSO) and/or LeFort I osteotomy (LFI) at a later age may be needed. LFI addresses the vertical and anterior-posterior defects (open bite); BSSO associated with the horizontal sliding osteotomy of the mandibular symphysis corrects the mandibular defect.

Goldenhar syndrome is a bilateral disease, which is characterized by a degree of agenesis and hypoplasia of the mandibular ramus, mandibular condyle, tragus, helix, antihelix, and temporomandibular joint (TMJ). The chin shows a degree of deviation and the margin of the mandible of the affected side is higher than the contralateral. The occlusion is Class II and the lower midline is displaced to the affected side. It should be treated by bilateral sagittal split osteotomy (BSSO) or mandibular osteodistraction based on the degree of severity and the experience of the surgeon. In case of severe deformity such as a serious joint involvement, BSSO may be indicated early around 9 years of age and it can be used with bone grafts for the restoration of the integrity of the ramus. However, the surgical correction of malocclusion occurs mostly in cases at the end of growth.

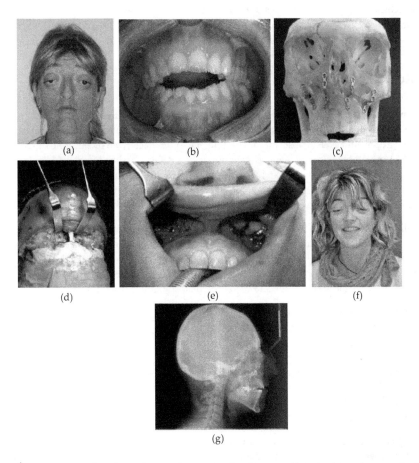

(a)   (b)   (c)

(d)   (e)   (f)

(g)

Figure 4. a) Preoperative frontal view showing the craniofacial malformation. b) Occlusal view demonstrating the open bite. c) Acrylic model with maxillary titanium plates adapted preoperatively to reproduce the LeFort I osteotomy. d) Intraoperative sequence showing the frontonasal surgical procedure. e) Intraoperative view of the LeFort I osteosynthesis. f) Postoperative photograph demonstrating an acceptable result. g) Postoperative radiographic control after surgery.

Apert and Crouzon syndrome are diseases characterized by synostosis of multiple sutures of the skull and the face; these diseases show a severe maxillary retrusion with a Class III malocclusion and open bite. The mandible has a normal shape. Common features are a narrow/high-arched palate, posterior bilateral crossbite, hypodontia, and crowding of teeth. The treatment begins early in the neonatal period if there are signs and symptoms of increased intracranial pressure. The first procedure is the advancement of the fronto-orbital complex to restore the cranial shape. The second step begins at around 6 years of age. The facial complex is osteotomized according to the Le Fort III line, eventually with a median osteotomy creating a facial bipartition. At the end of growth in many patients there is still a malocclusion. Surgical procedures depend on the defects; however, LFI is used to advance the maxilla, while correcting the open bite.[32] (Fig. 4 a-g)

7. Reverse facelift

The physiopathological basis of the aging face is not completely understood; however three factors contribute to the development of the aforementioned problem: soft tissue laxity, soft tissue atrophy and skeletal resorption. The aging face is characterized by multiple signs affecting the upper third (brow ptosis, excess of upper eyelid skin, forehead furrows, herniation of the orbital fat pad, glabellar frown lines); the middle third (accentuation of the parabuccal fat pad and development of the nasojugal fold) and the lower third (evidence of the labiomental fold, formation of the facial jowls and accentuation of the submental fat pad).[33-36]

Facelift procedures and fat grafting have been developed to restore a younger face and address the laxity and the atrophy of the soft tissue; the classic concept is that during life the force of gravity pulls the facial teguments down; facelift procedures pull the tissues up, both conventionally and more recently endoscopically. Moreover structural fat grafting accentuates the atrophic facial soft tissue and recreates the lost young tension.[37-39]

It is a common belief that the maxillofacial skeleton atrophies with the aging process, leading to a reduction of the facial height and depth; maxillary and mandibular bone resorption leads to a loss of support of the mouth and the nose. Maxillomandibular advancement (MMA) by orthognathic surgery restores the lost space dimension, providing projection to the cheeks, the jaws and the nose. In relation to the satisfactory esthetic results of orthognathic procedures performed on OSAS patients, the concept of "reverse face lift" started to arise. Maxillomandibular advancement is a very powerful tool to mask the physiological bone atrophy. It restores the space dimension by projecting the nose, the cheeks and the mouth.

The effect of bimaxillary manipulation on the facial soft tissue for dentofacial deformities has long been studied; conversely, the resultant facial changes of patients treated by MMA for OSAS has not been adequately described and the concept of "reverse face lift" has not been investigated in the scientific literature. Simultaneously MMA changes the skeletal framework of the face, improving soft tissue support and resulting in rejuvenation of the middle and the lower third of the face.

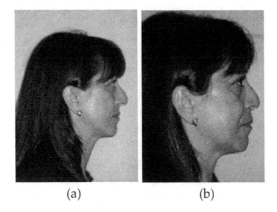

(a)   (b)

Figure 5. a) Lateral photograph of an aging face. b) Postoperative view after bimaxillary surgery of advancement showing the effects of reverse facelift.

Preoperative analysis of facial proportions with cephalometric measures, as performed with standard orthognathic cases, is of paramount importance before performing MMA for OSAS. Eventual unesthetic facial changes must be preoperatively discussed with the patient and the necessity of clockwise/counterclockwise rotation of the occlusal plane needs to be assessed in order to obtain a satisfactory result in terms of esthetics and functionality. Reverse facelift via bimaxillary advancements is a surgical procedure that may be combined with facelift procedures and structural fat grafting, can be indicated for a selected group of middle-aged patients, very motivated to an extreme rejuvenation. (Fig. 5a, b) [40-43]

8. Transgender surgery

Transsexualism is the extreme side of a wide spectrum of disorders called gender identity disorder (GID). It occurs when the anatomic gender of a person is opposite of his or her psychological gender. Epidemiological studies in the United States and Great Britain declare a prevalence of transsexualism of 1:50,000.

There are essential differences between male and female faces with regard to the skeleton and the soft tissues of the face. They have been extensively studied. The male forehead is flat and the supraorbital ridges are prominent. Females have a higher forehead with a more convex curvature. The orbits of the women are larger and higher. The zygomas of men are larger but less prominent. The mandible of men is larger, with a more prominent gonial angle and a rectangular chin.[44-46]

Gender reassignment requires both medical and surgical treatments. Hormonal therapy must be initiated early in the transgender process in order to change the physical features. The need for facial surgery to pass as a member of the other sex occurs in a significant percentage of transsexuals.

Facial feminization surgery (FFS) is referred as a group of surgical techniques devoted to change the features of a face from male to female. FFS was pioneered by Dr. Douglas Ousterhout from San Francisco, CA, USA in the 1980s. Facial feminization surgery (FFS) occurs more frequently than facial skeletal masculinisation and it is considered technically less demanding. Orthognathic surgery is a precious tool for a facial sexual reassignment surgical program.[47-50]Maxillary and mandibular osteotomies with clockwise rotation of the bimaxillary complex decreases the projection of both the chin and the mandibular angle region. Preoperative and postoperative orthodontic treatment is of paramount importance for the treatment plan. Le Fort I osteotomy (LFI) in association to a bilateral sagittal split osteotomy (BSSO) changes the geometry of the maxillo-mandibular complex.

The upper jaw can be placed forward in combination with a posterior vertical impaction. Although the mandibular angle does not change position with the BSSO and the dental occlusion remains unchanged, this clockwise rotation of the lower half of the face results in a more convex profile of the face with a less prominent chin which lead to a more feminine facial skeleton.

Orthognathic surgery is frequently associated with other procedures such as:

1. Mandibular angle reshaping to reduce the lower facial width;

2. Chin reduction to reshape the stigmata of the masculine chin;

3. Zygoma osteotomies with or without autogenous grafts/alloplastic implants to increase the mid-facial prominence;

4. Forehead recontouring to eliminate the frontal bossing;

5. Rhinoplasty to correct the stigmata of the male midface;

6. Browlift and scalp advancement to feminize the upper third of the face;

7. Lip lift, fat grafting and thyroid cartilage shave as ancillary procedures.[51] (Fig. 6 a-f)

9. Ethnic orthognathic surgery

There are certain differences in dental, skeletal, and soft-tissue facial morphology between Afro-American, Asian, Caucasian and Latin patients; orthognathic surgery must be adapted to each peculiar ethnic case. Meticulous planning ad careful execution of the osteotomies according to the preoperative surgical plan is essential to ensure an optimal outcome. Ethnic differences are related to the shape and the proportions of the skeletal framework, the soft tissue, and the texture of the skin. Individuals of all races, all over the world, desire to have an esthetically-ideal face. It is essential to understand the ethnic concepts of beauty for an optimal result.

Latin patients descend from the European immigrants and from the native population. For historical reasons, there is a Mongoloid component in their facial shape, making the same criteria of maxillofacial surgery applicable even for Asian populations. Because of similarities in anatomic characteristics such as skin thickness, wide bigonial angle and bimaxillary

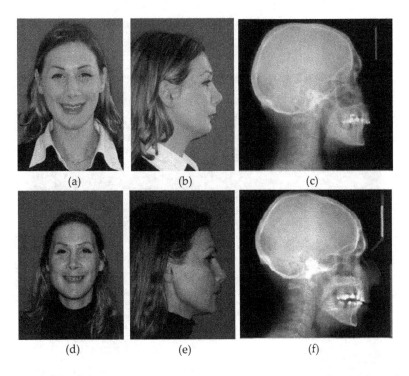

Figure 6. a) Preoperative frontal view. b) Preoperative lateral view. c) Preoperative radiographic examination. d) Post-operative smile after bimaxillary surgery. e) Lateral photograph demonstrating a feminine appearance. f) Teleradiography demonstrating orthognathic surgery.

protrusion, basic concepts can be applied even for some individuals of African origin. [52]A common characteristic is the protrusion of the dental arches, which lead to the projection of the lips with an acute nasolabial angle and the absence of the sublabial sulcus. The gingival display is excessive and the lip strain is exaggerated; the nasal spine appears receded and the paranasal areas appear depressed. The chin is located in a normal position; however it frequently appears receded because of the prominence of the dental arches; this feature augments the facial convexity. Standard surgical procedures include: Lefort I osteotomy to correct the midfacial deformities, bilateral sagittal split osteotomy to adapt the mandible, and subapical osteotomies to manage peculiar dento-alveolar discrepancies.

Surgical approach to alveolar protrusion requires careful planning and preoperative orthodontics. Model surgery needs to be performed in order to coordinate the dental arches after segmental surgery; finally intraoperative occlusal plates are fabricated. Two splints are necessary if bimaxillary protrusion is managed in a single stage as double-jaw surgery. Sophisticated studies about the vascularity of the maxilla and surgical refinements regarding the osteotomies lines have guaranteed predictable outcomes with minimal morbidity. Segmental osteotomies need to be performed without injuring adjacent teeth, while preserving the blood supply from the mucosa to the osseous segments.

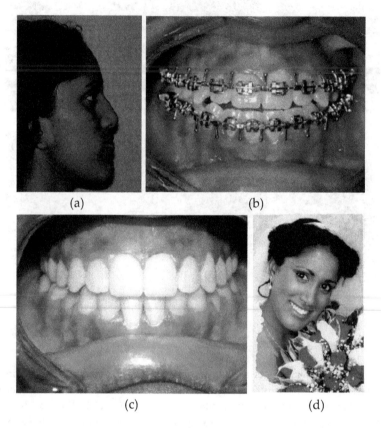

(a)   (b)

(c)   (d)

Figure 7. a) Preoperative frontal view. b) Preoperative malocclusion III class. c) Postoperative smile demonstrating a satisfactory result. d) Postoperative occlusal view.

The procedure can be managed by general or local anaesthesia. A vertical incision is performed on each side of the upper arch from the alveolus of the first premolar, which is extracted, toward to the vestibular sulcus. A segment of bone is removed from the palatine process and from the alveolar arch in order to displace the premaxilla backward. Osteosynthesis is performed with titanium plates and screws eventually associated to orthodontic bar.

Deformity of the mandibular dental arch is managed in a similar fashion. The incision is placed vertically in the mucosa from the first premolar toward the vestibular cul-de-sac. Then, subperiosteal dissection of the buccal and lingual cortex of the mandible is executed. One vertical osteotomy for each side of the arch is extended beyond the dental roots. Then, a horizontal osteotomy is made joining the aforementioned osteotomies. The excess of bone is resected. The segment is mobilized and with the occlusal bite in place osteosynthesis is done with plates and screws.

Orthognathic procedures for correcting skeletal deformities can be used in association with maxillary and mandibular osteotomies. Frequently, skeletal surgery is combined with adjunctive procedures such as: forehead lift, facelift, rhinoplasty and fat grafting to augment facial beauty.[53,54] (Fig. 7a–d)

10. Reoperative orthognathic surgery

Although orthognathic surgery is considered a routine procedure in the common practice of oral and maxillofacial surgery, problems can arise at any point of the orthodontic-surgical process: the preoperative diagnosis and planning, the orthodontic therapy and the surgical phase. Complications can be divided into: airway, vascular, neurologic, infectious, dental, skeletal and cosmetic. Complications which require reoperation can occur; problems must be careful identified and solved to obtain an optimal result in terms of esthetics and functionality.

A full description based on an extensive literature review regarding the incidence of the complications among the different orthognathic procedures is beyond the scope of this chapter. However, intraoperative and/or postoperative hemorrhage, hypoesthesia /anaesthesia of the trigeminal branches, lesion of the cranial nerves and the skull base, maxillary avascular and aseptic necrosis and bone or soft tissue infection can occur at any time even for the most experienced surgeon.

Reoperative orthognathic surgery is required when the results obtained after the initial treatment are not satisfactory in terms of esthetics or functionality. Complications which require reoperation can occur during the surgery, in the initial postoperative phase, and after weeks/ months from the initial treatment.

The proper position of the condyle in the glenoid fossa is a manoeuvre which tremendously affects the final dental and skeletal occlusion. Condylar sag can be classified as central, peripheral type I and peripheral type II from maxillary or mandibular surgery. Central condylar sag can occur if the condyle is positioned inferiorly in the glenoid fossa without bone contact with the fossa. After removal of the intraoperative maxillo-mandibular fixation (IMMF), the condyle will move superiorly, causing an anterior open bite if the problem is bilateral. If only 1 side is affected, the lower dental midline will move toward the affected side and the occlusion of the affected side will be class II.

Peripheral condylar sag type II occurs when excessive pressure is placed on the proximal segment during osteosynthesis which leads to a superolateral movement of the condyle. If it occurs bilaterally, the final occlusion will be a posterior open bite; if it occurs only on 1 side, the occlusion will be a posterior bite only on the affected side and the lower dental midline will move toward to the opposite side of the affected side.[55]

Central condylar sag may also occur after Le Fort I osteotomy. Condyles may be inferiorly distracted from the glenoid fossa due to posterior bony interference of the maxilla. When IMMF is applied, the mandible will rotate counter clockwise with the posterior teeth as a fulcrum. When IMMF is removed, a class II anterior open bite can result. This event can occur both intraoperatively or in the immediate postoperative period.

Late postoperative complications which require orthognathic surgery can be due to unexpected postoperative growth, idiopathic condylar resorption or peripheral condylar sagging type I. Unexpected late facial growth may take place months or years after the surgical procedure. This is a very challenging issue for the surgeon to determine if the mandibular growth continues and if it should be treated orthodontically or surgically.

Idiopathic condylar resorption is related to the effects of chronic excessive loading of the mandibular condyle. It affects bilaterally and symmetrically the condyle of women between the age of 15 and 30 years. The resorption is progressive and painless, leading to a gradual loss of the ramus height, with a class II anterior open bite. A technetium 99m bone scan will determine if the bone activity is active. Occlusion should be stable for a minimum of 1 year. Patients can be treated by means of orthognathic surgery or with replacement of the mandibular condyle with a total-joint temporomandibular joint prosthesis in cases of severe functional and esthetic problems.

Peripheral condylar sag type I occurs when excessive pressure is placed on the mandibular condyle during osteosynthesis of the fragments which lead to an inferiorly sliding of the condyle with bone contact. This provides stability to the occlusion, and the problem can not be identified at the time of surgery. Resorption of the lateral pole of the condyle can make the problem become apparent even months after surgery. This resorption will cause the condyle to slide superiorly into the fossa; the mandible will relapse posteriorly on the affected side.

Finally, after 6-12 months after surgery, any unsatisfactory esthetic results are analyzed and corrective surgery can be eventually scheduled for soft tissue problems (nasal, midface, lip esthetics) and hard tissue concerns (facial asymmetry, anteroposterior and vertical discrepancies).[56]

Author details

F. Arcuri[1*], M. Giarda[1], L. Stellin[1], A. Gatti[1], M. Nicolotti[1], M. Brucoli[1], A. Benech[1] and P. Boffano[2]

*Address all correspondence to: fraarcuri@libero.it

1 Department of Maxillo-Facial Surgery, Novara Major Hospital: University of Eastern Piedmont "Amedeo Avogadro", Novara, Italy

2 University of Turin, Italy

References

[1] Obwegeser, H. (1965). Surgery of the maxilla for the correction of prognathism. *Schweizerische Montatsschrift fur Zahnheilkunde*, 75, 365-74.

[2] Obwegeser, H. (1964). The indications for surgical correction of mandibular deformity by the sagittal splitting technique. *Br J Oral Surg*, 2, 157-71.

[3] Trauner, R., & Obwegeser, H. (1957). The surgical correction of mandibular prognathism and retrognathia with consideration of genioplasty: Part I. Surgical procedures to correct mandibular prognathism and reshaping of the chin. *Oral Surg*, 10, 667.

[4] Bell, W.H. (1977). Correction of maxillary excess by anterior maxillary osteotomy. A review of three basic procedures. *Oral Surg Oral Med Oral Pathol*, 43(3), 323-32.

[5] Lachard, J., Blanc, J. L., Lagier, J. P., Cheynet, F., Le Retraite, C., & Saban, Y. (1987). Köle's operation. *Rev Stomatol Chir Maxillofac*, 88(5), 306-10.

[6] Ermel, t., Hoffmann, J., Alfter, G., & Göz, G. (1999). Long-term stability of treatment results after upper jaw segmented osteotomy according to Schuchardt for correction of anterior open bite. *J Orofac Orthop*, 60(4), 236-45.

[7] Hebert, J. M., Kent, J. N., & Hinds, E. C. (1970). Correction of prognathism by intraoral vertical subcondylar osteotomy. *J Oral Surg*, 28, 651-665.

[8] Abubaker, A. O., & Sotereanos, G. C. (1991). Modified Le Fort I (Maxillary-Zygomatic) osteotomy: rationale, basis, and surgical technique. *J Oral Maxillofac Surg*, 49, 1089-1097.

[9] Keller, E.E, & Sather, A.H. (1990). Qadrangular Le Fort I osteotomy: surgical technique and review of 54 patients. *J Oral Maxillofac Surg*, 48, 2-11.

[10] Mc Ardle, N., Devereux, G., et al. (1999). Long term use of CPAP therapy for sleep apnea/hypopnea syndrome. *Am J Respir Crit Care Med*, 159, 1108-14.

[11] Lin, H. C., Friedman, M., Chang, H. W., & Gurpinar, B. (2008). The efficacy of multilevel surgery of upper airway in adults with obstructive sleep apnea/hypopnea syndrome. *Laryngoscope*, 118, 902-908.

[12] Fairburn, S. C., Waite, P. D., Vilos, G., et al. (2007). Three-dimensional changes in upper airways f patients with obstructive sleep apnea following maxillomandibular advancement. *J Oral Maxillofac Surg*, 65, 6-12.

[13] Lye, K. W., Waite, P. D., Meara, D., & Wang, D. (2008). Quality of life evaluation of maxillo-mandibular advancement surgery for treatment of obstructive sleep apnea. *J Oral Maxillofac Surg*, 66, 968-972.

[14] Holty, J. C., & Guilleminault, C. (2010). Maxillomandibular advancement for treatment of obstructive sleep apnea: a systematic review and meta analysis. *Sleep Med Rev*, 14, 287-297.

[15] Giarda, M., Brucoli, M., Arcuri, F., Braghiroli, A., Aluffi, P., & Benech, A. (2012). Proposal of a presurgical algorithm for patients affected by obstructive sleep apnea syndrome. *J Oral Maxillofac Surg*, Jan 27, Epub ahead of print.

[16] Branemark, P. I., Hansson, B. O., Adell, R., et al. (1977). Osseointegrated implants in the treatment of the edentulous jaw. Experience from a 10-year period. *Scand J Plast Reconstr Surg Suppl*, 16, 1-132.

[17] Albrektsson, T. (1988). A multicenter report on osseointegrated oral implants. *J Prosthet Dent*, 60, 75-84.

[18] Adell, R., Lekbolm, U., Rockier, B., et al. (1981 A). A 15-year study of osseointegrated implants in the treatment of the edentulous jaw. *Int J Oral Surg*, 10, 387-416.

[19] Sailer, H.F. (1989). A new method of inserting endosseous implants in totally atrophic maxillae. *J Craniomaxillofac Surg*, 30, 299-305.

[20] Cawood, J. I., & Stoelinga, P. J. (2000). International Research Group on Reconstructive Preprosthetic Surgery. Consensus report. *Int J Oral maxillofac Surg*, 29, 159-162.

[21] Malo, P., de Araujo, Nobre. M., & Lopes, A. (2007). The use of computer-guided flapless implant surgery and four implants placed in immediate function to support a fixed denture: preliminary results after a mean follow-up period of thirteen months. *J Prosthet Dent*, 97, S26-S34.

[22] Johansson, B., Friberg, B., & Nilson, H. (2009). Digitally planned, immediately loaded dental implants with prefabricated prostheses in the reconstruction of edentulous maxillae: a 1-year prospective, multicenter study. *Clin Implant Dent Relat Res*, 11, 194-200.

[23] Yerit, K. C., Martin, P., Guserl, U., Turhani, D., Schopper, C., Wanschitz, F., Wagner, A., Watzinger, F., & Ewers, R. (2004). Rehabilitation of the severely atrophied maxilla by horseshoe Le Fort I osteotomy (HLFO). *Oral Surg Oral Med Oral Pathol Oral Radiol Endod*, 97, 683-692.

[24] Yang, R. S., Salama, A. R., & Caccamese, J. F. (2011). Reoperative midface trauma. *Oral Maxillofac Surg Clin North Am*, 23(1), 31-45.

[25] Imola, MJ, Ducic, Y., & Adelson, R. T. (2008). The secondary correction of post-traumatic craniofacial deformities. *Otolaryngol Head Neck Surg*, 139(5), 654-60.

[26] Jones, T. A., Garg, T., & Monaghan, A. (2004). Removal of a deeply impacted mandibular third molar through a sagittal split ramus osteotomy approach. *Br J Oral Maxillofac Surg*, 42(4), 365-8.

[27] Scolozzi, P., Lombardi, T., & Jaques, B. (2007). Le Fort I Type Osteotomy and Man- dibular Sagittal Osteotomy as a Surgical Approach for Removal of Jaw Cysts. *J Oral Maxillofac Surg*, 65, 1419-1426.

[28] Scolozzi, P., Lombardi, T., & Jaques, B. (2004). Successful inferior alveolar nerve de- compression for dysesthesia following endodontic treatment: report of 4 cases treat- ed by mandibular sagittal osteotomy. *Oral Surg Oral Med Oral Pathol Oral Radiol Endod*, 97(5), 625-31.

[29] Girish, Rao. S., Sudhakara, Reddy. K., & Sampath, S. (2012). Lefort I access for juve- nile nasopharyngeal angiofibroma (JNA): a prospective series of 22 cases. *J Cranio- maxillofac Surg*, 40(2), e 54-8.

[30] Heliövaara, A., Ranta, R., Hukki, J., & Rintala, A. (2002). Skeletal stability of Le Fort I osteotomy in patients with isolated cleft palate and bilateral cleft lip and palate. *Int J Oral Maxillofac Surg*, 31(4), 358-63.

[31] Wolford, L. M., Cassano, D. S., Cottrell, D. A., El Deeb, M., Karras, S. C., & Gon- calves, J. R. (2008). Orthognathic surgery in the young cleft patient: preliminary study on subsequent facial growth. *J Oral Maxillofac Surg*, 66(12), 2524-36.

[32] Kahnberg, K. E., & Hagberg, C. (2010). Orthognathic surgery in patients with cranio- facial syndrome. I. A 5-year overview of combined orthodontic and surgical correc- tion. *J Plast Surg Hand Surg*, 44(6), 282-8.

[33] Arcuri, F, Brucoli, M, Benech, R, Giarda, M, & Benech, A. (2011). Maxillomandibular advancement in obstructive sleep apnea syndrome patients: a surgical model to in- vestigate reverse face lift. *J Craniofac Surg*, 22(6), 2148-52.

[34] Sherris, D. A., & Larrabee, W. F. Jr. (1996). Anatomic considerations in rhytidectomy. *Facial Plast Surg*, 12(3), 215-22.

[35] Ramirez, O.M. (2000). The central oval of the face: tridimensional endoscopic rejuve- nation. *Facial Plast Surg*, 16(3), 283-98.

[36] Coleman, S. R. (1998). Structural fat grafting. *Aesthet Surg J*, 18(5), 386-388.

[37] Arnett, G. W., & Gunson, M. J. (2010). Esthetic treatment planning for orthognathic surgery. *J Clin Orthod*, 44(3), 196-200.

[38] Hwang, S. J., Haers, P. E., Seifert, B., & Sailer, H. F. (2004). Non-surgical risk factors for condylar resorption after orthognathic surgery. *J Craniomaxillofac Surg*, 32(2), 103-11.

[39] Pessa, J. E., Zadoo, V. P., Mutimer, K. L., Haffner, C., Yuan, C., De Witt, A. I., & Gar- za, J. R. (1998). Relative maxillary retrusion as a natural consequence of aging: com- bining skeletal and soft-tissue changes into an integrated model of midfacial aging. *Plast Reconstr Surg*, 102(1), 205-12.

[40] Riley, R. W., Powell, N. B., & Guilleminault, C. (1993). Obstructive sleep apnea syndrome: A review of 306 consecutively treated surgical patients. *Otolaryngol Head Neck Surg*, 108, 117-25.

[41] Abramson, Z., Susarla, S., August, M., Troulis, M., & Kaban, L. (2010). Three-dimensional computed tomographic analysis of airway anatomy in patients with obstructive sleep apnea. *J Oral Maxillofac Surg*, 68(2), 354-62.

[42] Joss, C. U., Joss-Vassalli, I. M., Bergé, S. J., & Kuijpers-Jagtman, A. M. (2010). Soft tissue profile changes after bilateral sagittal split osteotomy for mandibular setback: a systematic review. *J Oral Maxillofac Surg*, 68(11), 2792-801.

[43] Jensen, A. C., Sinclair, P. M., & Wolford, L. M. (1992). Soft tissue changes associated with double jaw surgery. *Am J Orthod*, 101, 266.

[44] Shams, M. G., & Motamedi, M. H. (2009). Case report: feminizing the male face. *Eplasty*, 9, e2, Epub Jan 9.

[45] Cohen-Kettenis, P. T., & Gooren, L. J. (1999). Transsexualism: a review of etiology, diagnosis and treatment. *J Psychosom Res*, 46, 315-33.

[46] Hoenig, J., & Kenna, J. C. (1974). The prevalence of transsexualism in England and Wales. *Br J Psychiatry*, 124, 181-90.

[47] Monstrey, S., Hoebeke, P., Dhont, M., et al. (2001). Surgical therapy in transsexual patients: a multidisciplinary approach. *Acta Chir Belg*, 101, 200-9.

[48] Ousterhout, D.K. (1987). Feminization of the forehead: contour changing to improve female anesthetics. *Plast Reconstr Surg*, 79, 701.

[49] Mommaerts, M. Y., Abeloos, J. V. S., Calix, A. S., et al. (1995). The "sandwich" zygomatic osteotomy: technique, indications and clinical results. *J Craniomaxiliofac Surg*, 23, 12-9.

[50] Ousterhout, D.K. (2011). Dr. Paul Tessier and facial skeletal masculinization. *Ann Plast Surg*, 67(6), 10-5.

[51] Becking, A. G., Tuinzing, D. B., Hage, J. J., & Gooren, L. J. (1996). Facial corrections in male to female transsexuals: a preliminary report on 16 patients. *J Oral Maxillofac Surg*, 54(4), 413-418.

[52] Beugre, J. B., Sonan, N. K., Beugre-Kouassi, A. M., & Djaha, F. (2007). Comparative cephalometric study of three different ethnic groups of black Africa with normal occlusion. *Odontostomatol Trop*, 30(117), 34-44.

[53] Chew, M.T. (2006). Spectrum and management of dentofacial deformities in a multiethnic Asian population. *Angle Orthod*, 76(5), 806-9.

[54] Clemente-Panichella, D., Suzuki, S., & Cisneros, G. J. (2000). Soft to hard tissue movement ratios: orthognathic surgery in a Hispanic population. *Int J Adult Orthodon Orthognath Surg*, 15(4), 255-64.

[55] Reyneke, J.P. (2011). Reoperative orthognathic surgery. *Oral Maxillofac Surg Clin North Am*, 23(1), 73-92.

[56] Chow, L. K., Singh, B., Chiu, W. K., & Samman, N. (2007). Prevalence of postoperative complications after orthognathic surgery: a 15 -year review. *J Oral Maxillofac Surg*, 65(5), 984-92.

Chapter 6

Soft-tissue Response in Orthognathic Surgery Patients Treated by Bimaxillary Osteotomy – Cephalometry Compared with 2-D Photogrammetry

Jan Rustemeyer

Additional information is available at the end of the chapter

1. Introduction

During recent decades, orthognathic surgery has become widely accepted as the preferred method of correcting moderate-to-severe skeletal deformities including facial esthetics. Recognition of esthetic factors and prediction of the final facial profile play an increasingly important role in orthognathic treatment planning, since the facial profile produced by orthognathic surgery is highly significant for patients [1-3]. Many studies have attempted to evaluate the relationship between hard-tissue surgery and its effect on the overlying soft tissue for predicting facial changes [4-6]. Three-dimensional (3-D) imaging techniques, including computer tomography, video imaging, laser scanning, morphanalysis, 3-D sonography, and, recently, 3-D photogrammetry [7-13] have been developed to highlight the relationship between hard- and soft-tissue movements, but details of this relationship, particularly in the vertical direction, have varied and not been fully clarified [14]. However, the assessment of visible volume changes with an optical 3-D sensor can be carried out with considerable accuracy and provides the opportunity to complete cephalometric analysis in cases of midfacial distractions and asymmetric craniofacial situations [15].

For routine orthognathic surgery cases, cephalometry and 2-D photogrammetry are common and less expensive tools that may have the potential to analyze and predict the resulting profile. However, it is remarkable that no recent report offers a comparison between both conventional methods of indirect anthropometry. Therefore, the objective of this study was to assess the facial soft-tissue response in skeletal Class II and III patients treated by bimaxillary orthognathic surgery both cephalometrically and with 2-D photogrammetry and to compare their ability to predict postoperative outcomes. Hence, the relevant questions were whether both methods have the capacity to complement one another or not and in which cases.

2. Patients and methods

Patients` sample

Twenty-eight patients who had undergone bimaxillary surgery for a Class II relationship (mean age, 24.5 ± 4.9 years; 18 females, 10 males) and 33 patients who had undergone bimaxillary surgery for a Class III relationship (mean age, 23.4 ± 3.7 years; 20 females, 13 males) were selected from adult treatment records. Bimaxillary surgery consisted of LeFort I osteotomy with maxillary advancement and/or impaction and bilateral sagittal split ramus osteotomy carried out for mandibular setback or advancement. Setback of the maxilla was not done. No additional surgical procedures were performed on the midface or chin, such as infraorbital augmentation, distraction, rhinoplasty, or genioplasty. Exclusion criteria to avoid any bias were patients' findings that exceeded routine orthognathic planning. These were patients with an anterior open bite of more than 1 cm, facial asymmetry with occlusal cants in the frontal plane, midline deviations and mandibular border asymmetry, matured cleft lip and palate, severe congenital facial deformity, and posttraumatic deformity.

All subjects had available both a lateral cephalogram and a lateral photogram in the natural head position (NHP) taken before orthodontic appliances were applied and nine months postsurgery, after removal of the orthodontic appliances and osteosynthesis materials (median follow-up: 9.4 ± 0.6 month).

Lateral cephalometry

Subjects were positioned in the cephalostat (Orthoceph, Siemens AG, Munich, Germany), and then the head holder was adjusted until the ear rods could be positioned into the ears without moving the patient. All radiographs were taken in the NHP with teeth together and lips in repose and with a metric ruler in front of the midfacial vertical line. No occipital supplement was used. According to cephalometric standards, the film distance to the X-ray tube was fixed at 150 cm and the film distance to the midsagittal plane of the patient's head at 18 cm.

Tracings were done for all cephalograms. After loading the cephalogram into a PC, the ruler was used to size the cephalogram image in the software program (Adobe Photoshop version 7.0, Adobe Systems, San Jose, CA, USA), so that 1 mm on the rule represented 1 mm of actual scale (life-size) in the software program. The landmarks were identified manually by a single examiner using the photographic software. Soft- and hard-tissue landmarks of the cephalograms were traced using a modified version of the analysis of Legan and Burstone [16] and Lew et al [17] (Figs. 1 and 2). Therefore, the horizontal reference line was constructed by raising a line 7° from sella-nasion, and a line perpendicular to this at nasion was used as the vertical reference line. Movement of hard- and soft-tissue landmarks from pre- to postsurgery was measured in millimeters to the horizontal and vertical reference lines. The corresponding angles were constructed and measured in degrees in the presurgical and postsurgical cephalograms. Differences were recorded as the surgical change.

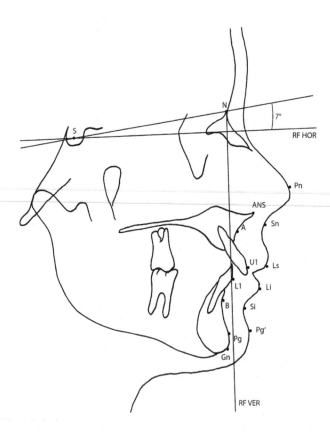

Figure 1. Hard and soft tissue landmarks and reference lines for tracing cephalograms.(N) = Nasion; (S) = Sella; (A) = Point A; (B) = Point B; (L1) = Lower incisor, (U1) = Upper incisor; (Gn) = Gnathion; (Pg) = Pogonium); (ANS) = Anterior nasal spine; (Pn) = Pronasale; (Sn) = Subnasale; (Ls) = Labrale superius; (Li) = Labrale inferius; (Si) = Labiomental sulcus; (Pg`) = Soft tissue pogonion; (RF HOR) = Horizontal reference line; (RF VER) = Vertical reference line.

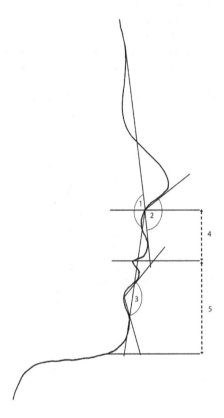

Figure 2. Soft-tissue angles and distances for tracing cephalograms and photograms. 1: Facial Convexity; 2: Nasolabial angle; 3: Labiomental angle; 4: Upper lip length; 5: Lower lip length.

2-D photogrammetry

Subjects were asked to sit on a chair in front of a pale blue background, maintain a straight back, and look straight ahead with a relaxed facial expression and eyes fully open, lips gently closed, and not smiling. A neck holder was then adjusted to help the subjects fix their NHP. For reproducibility, a simple, indirect light source on the ceiling was used, consisting of four 60-W fluorescent tubes to eliminate undesirable shadows from the contours of the facial profile. The subjects' faces were photographed in right lateral view, together with a metric scaled ruler in front of the midfacial vertical line (true vertical, TV). A high-resolution digital camera with a flash (Canon 450D, Tokyo, Japan) was firmly mounted on a photo stand 1 m in front of the subject. All photographs were taken at 2048 × 1536 pixels resolution and saved in JPEG file format. Images were stored on the PC's hard drive and then transferred into the photographic software program. The lateral photographs were adjusted to life-size according to the cephalogram adjustment as above. Soft-tissue landmarks, distances, and angles were traced with the tools of the software. Additionally, TV on nasion and true horizontal (TH, perpendicular to TV through the tragus) were constructed as reference lines for horizontal and vertical landmark movements. Pre- and postsurgical distances of each landmark toward reference lines were measured and differences were recorded as the vertical and horizontal surgical change, respectively (Figs. 2 and 3).

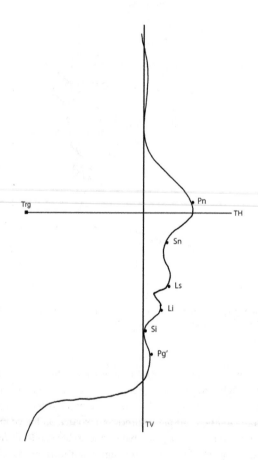

Figure 3. Soft- tissue landmarks and reference lines for tracing photograms.

(TV) = True Vertical; (TH) = True Horizontal; (Trg) = Tragus. Further abbreviations as given in Table 1.

Statistics and reliability of measurements

The collected data were subjected to statistical analysis using the PASW statistical software package, version 18.0 (SPSS, Chicago, IL, USA). Differences between groups were evaluated using the paired *t* test. Results were considered significant if $p< 0.05$ and highly significant if $p< 0.01$. Pearson`s correlation analysis was used to assess the degree of correlation between soft- and hard tissue changes. The adjusted coefficient of determination (Adj R^2) was used to assess the predictability of landmark movements (ranging from 0 = no prediction possible to 1 = accurate prediction possible).

Reliability of measurements was determined by randomly selecting 10 cephalograms and 10 lateral photograms to repeat the tracings by a second senior examiner. The method error was calculated using the formula $\sqrt{\sum (x_1-x_2)^2}/2n$ in which X_1 was the first measurement, X_2, the second measurement, and n, the number of repeated records. All respective values of method error calculation for the linear measurements ranged between 0.32 and 0.48 mm for cephalometry and between 0.35 and 0.51 mm for 2-D photogrammetry, for angular measurements between 1.4° and 5.2° and between 1.6° and 4.9°, respectively. Significant differences between the reliability of photogrammetry and cephalometry could not be obtained.

3. Results

General findings

Significant differences between females and males could not be obtained cephalometrically or photogrammetrically, nor with respect to angular or distance measurements, pre- or postoperative, nor landmark movements. Therefore, gender was not considered further.

Hard-tissue angles assessed by cephalometry changed significantly from pre- to postsurgery in Class II and Class III patients (SNA, p Class II = 0.041, p Class III = 0.015; SNB, p Class II = 0.009, p Class III = 0.008; ANB, p Class II = 0.016, p Class III<0.001; NAPg, p Class II = 0.043, p Class III< 0.001).

Soft tissue angles and distances

Significant differences between pre- and postsurgical measurements could be found for facial convexity, labiomental angle, and lower lip length by cephalometric and photogrammetric analyses (Table 1). Pre- to postsurgical changes of facial convexity in Class III patients and changes of lower lip length and labiomental angle in Class II patients revealed high significance ($p< 0.01$, Fig. 4). No significant changes from pre- to postsurgery could be found for the nasolabial angle or upper lip length.

		Photogrammetry			Cephalometry		
		presurgery	postsurgery		presurgery	postsurgery	
Parameter	Class	Mean ± SD	Mean ± SD	p	Mean ± SD	Mean ± SD	p
Facial convexity (°)	II	159.1 ± 4.8	165.9 ± 5.1	0.023*	159.8 ± 2.3	163.5 ± 3.4	0.015*
	III	178.8 ± 5.9	172.1 ± 6.1	<0.001**	178.8 ± 5.9	170.8 ± 7.3	<0.001**
Nasolabial angle (°)	II	111.2 ± 7.4	109.2 ± 9.2	0.671	111.4 ± 10.1	111.2 ± 7.5	0.976
	III	105.4 ± 12.4	104.6 ± 13.3	0.835	102.1 ± 14.2	103.2 ± 14.7	0.804
Labiomental angle (°)	II	119.1 ± 11.9	135.9 ± 9.8	0.013*	120.8 ± 7.4	134.2 ± 9.9	0.021*
	III	132.8 ± 14.6	121.1 ± 15.8	0.013*	127.4 ± 12.9	115.5 ± 13.8	0.004**
Upper lip length (mm)	II	13.5 ± 1.7	13.9 ± 1.3	0.621	13.9 ± 1.9	13.8 ± 1.9	0.533
	III	12.4 ± 1.6	13.1 ± 1.6	0.134	12.5 ± 2.1	13.1 ± 1.8	0.317
Lower lip length (mm)	II	24.7 ± 3.1	30.5 ± 3.3	0.006**	29.9 ± 2.3	29.9 ± 2.3	0.007**
	III	31.2 ± 3.4	28.8 ± 3.9	0.029*	31.6 ± 2.9	28.4 ± 2.7	0.003**

Table 1. *significant at the level p < 0.05, ** significant at the level p < 0.01. Pre- and postsurgical measurements of soft-tissue angles and distances.

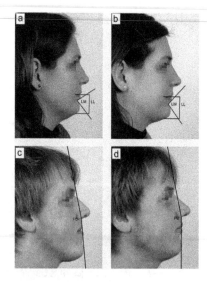

Figure 4. Screenshots of traced lateral photograms. Pre- to postsurgical changes of lower lip length (LL) and labiomental angle (LM) in Class II patients (a = presurgery, b = postsurgery) and changes of facial convexity (FC) in Class III patients (c = presurgery, d = postsurgery) revealed high significance.

Soft-tissue landmarks

Dimension	Landmark	Class	Photogrammetry Movement Mean ± SD	Cephalometry Movement Mean ± SD	p
Horizontal	Pn	II	0.9 ± 0.8	0.6 ± 0.5	0.251
		III	1.4 ± 2.6	1.1 ± 0.9	0.761
	Sn	II	2.1 ± 0.8	2.2 ± 0.9	0.883
		III	2.4 ± 1.6	1.2 ± 3.1	0.784
	Ls	II	2.5 ± 0.5	2.3 ± 1.7	0.831
		III	2.2 ± 1.6	1.1 ± 2.5	0.874
	Li	II	2.5 ± 0.8	2.2 ± 1.3	0.441
		III	-3.2 ± 2.1	-4.8 ± 3.1	0.376
	Si	II	2.7 ± 0.5	2.3 ± 0.8	0.421
		III	-5.4 ± 2.9	-5.9 ± 3.4	0.776
	PG`	II	2.5 ± 1.1	3.3 ± 1.2	0.232
		III	-6.8 ± 4.1	-6.1 ± 4.3	0.769
Vertical	Pn	II	0.1 ± 0.8	0.3 ± 0.5	0.451
		III	0.6 ± 1.1	0.4 ± 0.5	0.736
	Sn	II	0.2 ± 0.9	-0.2 ± 0.7	0.525
		III	0.6 ± 0.4	0.2 ± 0.4	0.688
	Ls	II	-0.5 ± 1.6	0.2 ± 0.9	0.418
		III	1.2 ± 0.8	1.4 ± 2.5	0.807
	Li	II	-0.6 ± 0.8	0.3 ± 1.2	0.187
		III	1.2 ± 2.1	2.5 ± 2.6	0.411
	Si	II	-1.3 ± 1.6	-0.2 ± 1.3	0.205
		III	1.8 ± 1.9	2.6 ± 1.9	0.283
	PG`	II	-1.2 ± 0.8	-0.7 ± 0.7	0.204
		III	1.4 ± 1.8	1.8 ± 2.3	0.199

Table 2. Pre- to postsurgical movements (mm) of soft-tissue landmarks in horizontal and vertical dimensions assessed by photogrammetry and cephalometry.

The measurements of pre- to postsurgical soft-tissue landmark movements did not differ significantly between photogrammetry and cephalometry (Table 2). In Class III patients, the greatest movements were found photogrammetrically and cephalometrically for Pg' in the horizontal and for Si in the vertical dimension. In Class II patients, Si movements assessed by photogrammetry and Pg' movements assessed by cephalometry revealed the greatest movements in both horizontal and vertical directions.

Correlations between soft- and hard-tissue changes

Significant correlations between soft- and hard-tissue changes (Table 3) occurred cephalometrically only in Class III patients. Highly significant correlations were found between facial convexity and SNB, ANB, and NAPg and between lower lip length and SNB, ANB, and NAPg. Photogrammetrically significant correlations occurred in Class II patients for labiomental angle and SNB, ANB, and NAPg and in Class III patients for facial convexity and NAPg; for nasolabial angle and SNA; and for lower lip length and NAPg. Significant correlations for both Class II and III patients could be shown between lower lip length and ANB.

	Parameters[a]	Class	SNA	SNB	ANB	NAPg
Cephaloametry	Facial convexity	II	ns	ns	ns	ns
		III	ns	0.003**	<0.001**	<0.001**
	Upper lip lenght	II	ns	ns	ns	ns
		III	ns	ns	0.032*	0.010*
	Lower lip lenght	II	ns	ns	ns	ns
		III	ns	0.002**	<0.001**	0.003**
Photogrammetry	Facial convexity	II	ns	ns	ns	ns
		III	ns	ns	ns	0.036*
	Nasolabial angle	II	ns	ns	ns	ns
		III	0.034*	ns	ns	ns
	Labiomental angle	II	ns	0.038*	0.037*	0.030*
		III	ns	ns	ns	ns
	Lower lip lenght	II	ns	ns	0.027*	ns
		III	ns	ns	0.032*	0.047*

Table 3. [a] only parameters revealing at least one significance were considered ns: indicates not significant; * significant at the level $p < 0.05$, ** significant at the level $p < 0.01$. Significance of correlations between soft- and hard-tissue changes

Correlations of hard- and soft-tissue movements between pre- and postoperative corresponding landmarks in the horizontal and vertical planes revealed significance for both cephalometry and 2-D photogrammetry in Class II and III patients (Table 4). Correlations could be found for both methods between Sn and A, Si and B, and Pg' and Pg in the horizontal plane for Class II and III patients. In the vertical plane for Class II patients, correlations could be shown cephalometrically only for Sn and A, and photogrammetrically only for Pg′ and Pg. In Class III patients, cephalometry and 2-D photogrammetry revealed both significant correlations between vertical movements of Sn and A, Ls and U1, and Pg′ and Pg. In cases of significant correlation, Adj R^2 was above the 0.7 level, representing a satisfactory accuracy for prediction.

Soft tissue parameter[a]	Hard tissue parameter[a]	Class	$p_{Sceph; H}$	Adj. R^2	$p_{Sphoto; H}$	Adj. R^2
Horizontal						
Sn	A	II	0.046*	0.717	0.011*	0.792
		III	0.044*	0.718	0.010*	0.891
Si	B	II	0.023*	0.707	0.038*	0.725
		III	0.034*	0.762	0.030*	0.778
Pg′	Pg	II	0.032*	0.752	0.015*	0.757
		III	0.010*	0.894	0.044*	0.720
Vertical						
Sn	A	II	0.036*	0.732	ns	0.121
		III	0.043*	0.721	0.016*	0.821
Ls	U1	II	ns	0.044	ns	0.044
		III	0.044*	0.721	0.018*	0.701
Pg′	Pg	II	ns	0.183	0.041*	0.712
		III	0.010*	0.889	0.030*	0.782

Table 4. [a] only parameters revealing at least one significance were considered. $p_{Sceph; H}$: significance of correlation between *cephalometrically* assessed soft- tissue landmark movement and corresponding hard-tissue landmark movement. $p_{Sphoto; H}$: significance of correlation between *photogrammetrically* assessed soft-tissue landmark movement and corresponding hard-tissue landmark movement. Adj. R^2: adjusted coefficient of determination. ns: indicates not significant; * significant at the level $p < 0.05$. Significances between hard- and soft-tissue landmark movement correlations .

Soft-to-hard tissue movement ratios

Soft-to-hard tissue movement ratios in the horizontal and vertical planes for corresponding landmarks displayed a soft-tissue response following hard-tissue movement (Table 5). No significant difference could be obtained between cephalometry and 2-D photogrammetry with respect to the soft- to hard-tissue movement ratios.

Soft- tissue parameter (S)	Hard- tissue parameter (H)	Class	Ratio S(ceph): H	Ratio S(photo): H
Horizontal				
Pn	ANS	II	0.33	0.73
		III	0.25	0.35
Sn	A	II	1.83	1.73
		III	0.39	0.59
Ls	U1	II	1.11	1.76
		III	0.27	0.60
Li	L1	II	0.88	1.09
		III	0.03	0.56
Si	B	II	1.27	1.35
		III	1.20	1.13
Pg`	Pg	II	1.13	1.09
		III	0.98	1.15
Vertical				
Pn	ANS	II	0.33	0.33
		III	0.40	0.60
Sn	A	II	0.06	0.03
		III	0.20	0.80
Ls	U1	II	0.25	0.35
		III	0.60	0.80
Li	L1	II	0.25	0.15
		III	0.33	0.07
Si	B	II	0.25	0.37
		III	1.37	0.83
Pg`	Pg	II	0.33	0.57
		III	1.49	0.57

Table 5. Soft-to-hard tissue movement ratios in horizontal and vertical dimensions for corresponding landmarks .

4. Discussion

The results of this study showed that maxillary and mandibular movements with bimaxillary osteotomy were effective on soft tissues both in vertical and horizontal directions, and they improved facial convexity to approximate esthetic norms. Arnett and Bergman [18,19] described the facial profile according to the angle of facial convexity in Class I (165°–175°), Class II (<165°), and Class III profiles (> 175°). Following this classification, in our study postsurgical Class I facial convexity was achieved in Class II and III patients and was assessed by 2-D photogrammetry as well as by cephalometry. However, cephalometric and photogrammetric changes of the labiomental angle could be obtained only in Class II patients. Fernández-Riveiro et al [20] found that the labiomental angle should be evaluated with caution because of its high method error and variability. In this study as well, photogrammetrically and cephalometrically defined labiomental angle measurements revealed the highest variability of all measurements.

Whereas horizontal movement of soft-tissue landmarks in Class II and III patients—with the exception of labrale superius and inferius—were strongly correlated cephalometrically and 2-D photogrammetrically with hard-tissue landmark movements, vertical movements of landmarks were mostly hard to predict. One reason might be that vertical mandibular movements in our patients were only minimal and beneath the capability of cephalometric and 2-D photogrammetric analyses, since patients with massive vertical deficits were excluded to avoid any bias in this study. Accordingly, Lin and Kerr [21] also found in their cohort that these may account for the increased difficulty in accurately predicting a change in the vertical dimension. In comparison, in the study of Nkenke et al. [15] using optical 3-D images for analysing soft-tissue advancement in patients undergoing midfacial distraction at 6 and 24 months postsurgically, means of vertical advancement of Sn (1.0 ± 1.0 mm; 0.4 ± 0.9 mm, respectively) and labrale superius (0.4 ± 1.1 mm; -0.2 ± 0.5 mm, respectively) were within the scope of the data assessed in this study by 2-D photogrammetry and cephalometry for Class II and III patients. Hence, adequate accuracy of determination of vertical movements could be achieved with both methods in this study and referring to the study of Nkenke et al. [15], the level of validity is acceptable. However, further studies are warranted to evaluate the concept of vertical changes in patients with extensive vertical discrepancies.

Findings in this study suggest that cephalometric and 2-D photogrammetric analyses complement one another in predicting soft-tissue changes in orthodontic surgery patients. For the combination of both methods, at least one parameter for the maxilla (Sn-A) and one for the mandible (Pg'-Pg) became predictable for the vertical dimension with an acceptable adjusted coefficient of determination. Special attention should be given to soft-tissue changes in Class II patients, which cephalometrically revealed no significant correlation with hard-tissue angular changes, whereas correlations could be obtained with 2-D photogrammetry. We therefore recommend supplementary 2-D photogrammetry for evaluating soft- to hard-tissue changes and cephalometric prediction, especially in Class II patients.

Previous cephalometric findings have shown mandibular skeletal movement for the soft-tissue chin at a ratio of between 0.9:1 and 1:1 [22,23]. The results of this study support this historical observations cephalometrically as well as 2-D-photogrammetrically for Class II and Class III patients. However, the labrale inferius (Li) in our study responded at a ratio of 0.88:1 cephalometrically and 1.09:1 photogrammetrically to the corresponding hard-tissue movements in the horizontal plane in Class II patients, but only at ratios of 0.03:1 and 0.56:1 in Class III patients, respectively. This is cephalometrically much lower than the ratio found in other investigations in Class III patients, which ranged from 0.6:1 to 0.75:1 [22, 23]. In comparison, with 2-D photogrammetry the lower border of this range was nearly reached.

Standard-error calculation suggests that standards presented in this study for cephalometry and 2-D photogrammetry set-ups are ready for routine evaluation of soft-tissue changes after orthognathic surgery. However, all ratios presented in this study and in the literature suggest that even a mathematically accurate prediction may involve bias [24]. This means that prediction and soft- to hard-tissue movement ratios must be evaluated on an individual basis and that they depend at least partly on the experience of the surgeon in his or her hand-setting of the maxilla during bimaxillary surgery. Furthermore, various types of operations—as well as the morphology of the anatomic structures—must be considered in predicting the outcome of facial surgery [25]. In comparison to data reported in another study from Nkenke et al. [26] using pre- and postsurgical 3-D facial surface images in patients undergoing LeFort I osteotomy, advancements of Sn and Ls were within the range of the results obtained in this study for horizontal movements of these parameters assessed with cephalometry and 2-D photogrammetry. Furthermore, the ratio of advancement between labrale superius and incision superius reported by Nkenke et al. [26] was 80 ± 94 % and comparable with our findings. In accordance to the ratios of vertical advancement and referring to the method of Nkenke et al. [26] again, validity of at least this ratio of horizontal advancement is adequate in our study. However, the 3-D facial surface images analysis possesses moreover the ability to predict volume increases or decreases especially in the malar- midface region and could therefore improve the predictability of esthetic soft tissue results. Future studies may reveal which orthognathic surgery cases are best suited for 3-D imaging techniques. The data of this study might be helpful.

5. Conclusion

This study revealed that cephalometry and 2-D photogrammetry provide the option to complement one another to enhance accuracy in predicting soft-tissue changes in orthodontic surgery, especially in Class II patients.

Acknowledgements

We gratefully acknowledge Ilknur Tetik, B.A., School of Architecture, Bremen, Germany, for her contribution to photogrammetric set-up.

Author details

Jan Rustemeyer*

Address all correspondence to: janrustem@gmx.de

Department of Oral and Maxillofacial Surgery, Klinikum Bremen-Mitte, School of Medicine
of the University of Göttingen, Germany

The authors declare they have no conflict of interest.

References

[1] Jacobson, A. (1984). Psychological aspects of dentofacial esthetics and orthognathic
     surgery. *Angle Orthod*, 54, 18-35.

[2] Kiyak, H. A., West, R. A., Hohl, T., & Mc Neill, R. W. (1982). The psychological im-
     pact of orthognathic surgery: a 9-month follow-up. *Am J Orthod*, 81, 404-412.

[3] Rustemeyer, J., Eke, Z., & Bremerich, A. (2010). Perception of omprovement after or-
     thognathic surgery: the important variables affecting patient satisfaction. *Oral Maxil-
     lofac Surg*, 14, 155-162.

[4] Chou, J. I., Fong, H. J., Kuang, S. H., Gi, L. Y., Hwang, F. Y., Lai, Y. C., Chang, R. C.,
     & Kao, S. Y. (2005). A retrospective analysis of the stability and relapse of soft and
     hard tissue change after bilateral sagittal split osteotomy for mandibular setback of
     64 Taiwanese patients. *J Oral Maxillofac Surg*, 63, 355-361.

[5] Enacar, A., Taner, T., & Toroglu, S. (1999). Analysis of soft tissue profile changes as-
     sociated with mandibular setback and double-jaw surgeries. *Int J Adult Orthod Or-
     thognath Surg*, 14, 27-35.

[6] Koh, C. H., & Chew, M. T. (2004). Predictability of soft tissue profile changes follow-
     ing bimaxillary surgery in skeletal Class III Chinese patients. *J Oral Maxillofac Surg*,
     62, 1505-1509.

[7] McCance, A. M., Moss, J. P., Fright, W. R., & Linney, A. D. (1997). Three-dimensional
     analysis technique-Part 3: Color-coded system for three-dimensional measurement of
     bone and ratio of soft tissue to bone: the analysis. *Cleft Palate Craniofac J*, 34, 52-57.

[8] Nanda, R. S., Ghosh, J., & Bazakidou, E. (1996). Three-dimensional facial analysis us-
     ing a video imaging system. *Angle Orthod*, 66, 181-188.

[9] Moss, J. P., Mc Cance, A. M., Fright, W. R., Linney, A. D., & James, D. R. (1994). A
     three-dimensional soft tissue analysis of fifteen patients with class II, division I mal-
     occlusions after bimaxillary surgery. *Am J Orthod Dentofac Orthop*, 105, 430-437.

[10] Rabey, G. (1971). Craniofacial morphanalysis. *Proc R Soc Med*, 64, 103-111.

[11] Hell, B. (1995). 3D sonography. *Int J Oral Maxillofac Surg*, 4, 84-89.

[12] Deli, R., Di Gioia, E., Galantucci, L. M., & Percoco, G. (2010). Automated landmark extraction for orthodontic measurement of faces using the 3-camera photogrammetry methodology. *J Craniofac Surg*, 21, 87-93.

[13] Plooij, J. M., Swennen, G. R., Rangel, F. A., Maal, T. J., Schutyser, F. A., Bronkhorst, E. M., Kuijpers-Jagtman, A. M., & Bergé, S. J. (2009). Evaluation of reproducibility and reliability of 3D soft tissue analysis using 3D stereophotogrammetry. *Int J Oral Maxillofac Surg*, 38, 267-273.

[14] Okudaira, M., Kawamoto, T., Ono, T., & Moriyama, K. (2008). Soft-tissue changes in association with anterior maxillary osteotomy: a pilot study. *Oral Maxillofac Surg*, 12, 131-138.

[15] Nkenke, E., Langer, A., Laboureux, X., Benz, M., Maier, T., Kramer, M., Häusler, G., Kessler, P., Wiltfang, J., & Neukam, F. W. (2003). Validation of in vitro assessment of facial soft-tissue volumne changes and clinical application in midfacial distraction: a technical report. *Plast Reconstr Surg*, 112, 367-380.

[16] Legan, H. L., & Burstone, C. l. (1980). Soft tissue cephalometric analysis for orthognathic surgery. 38, 744-751.

[17] Lew, K. K., Low, F. C., Yeo, J. F., & Loh, H. S. (1990). Evaluation of soft tissue profile following intraoral ramus osteotomy in Chinese adults with mandibular prognathism. *Int J Adult Orthodon Orthognath Surg*, 5, 189-197.

[18] Arnett, G. W., & Bergman, R. T. (1993). Facial keys to orthodontic diagnosis and treatment planning. Part I. *Am J Orthod Dentofacial Orthop*, 103, 299-312.

[19] Arnett, G. W., & Bergman, R. T. (1993). Facial keys to orthodontic diagnosis and treatment planning. Part II. *Am J Orthod Dentofacial Orthop*, 103, 395-411.

[20] Fernández-Riveiro, P., Smyth-Chamosa, E., Suárez-Quintanilla, A., & Suárez-Cunqueiro, A. (2003). Angular photogrammetric analysis of the soft tissue facial profile. *Eur J Orthod*, 25, 393-399.

[21] Lin, S. S., & Kerr, W. J. (1998). Soft and hard tissue changes in Class III patients treated by bimaxillary surgery. *Eur J Orthod*, 20, 25-33.

[22] Hershey, H. G., & Smith, L. H. (1974). Soft-tissue profile change associated with surgical correction of the prognathic mandible. *Am J Orthod*, 65, 483-502.

[23] Lines, P. A., & Steinhäuser, E. W. (1974). Soft tissue changes in relationship to movement of hard structures in orthognathic surgery: a preliminary report. *J Oral Surg*, 32, 891-896.

[24] Marşan, G., Cura, N., & Emekli, U. (2009). Soft and hard tissue changes after bimaxillary surgery in Turkish female Class III patients. *J Craniomaxillofac Surg*, 37, 8-17.

[25] Moss, J. P., Grindrod, S. R., Linney, A. D., Arridge, S. R., & James, D. (1988). A computer system for the interactive planning and prediction of maxillofacial surgery. *Am J Orthod Dentofac Orthop*, 94, 469-475.

[26] Nkenke, E., Vairaktaris, E., Kramer, M., Schlegel, A., Holst, A., Hirschfelder, U., Wiltfang, J., Neukam, F. W., & Stamminger, M. (2008). Three-dimensional analysis of changes of the malar-midfacial region after LeFort I osteotomy and maxillary advancement. *Oral Maxillofac Surg*, 12, 5-12.

Chapter 7

Corticotomy and Miniplate Anchorage for Treating Severe Anterior Open-Bite: Current Clinical Applications

Mehmet Cemal Akay

Additional information is available at the end of the chapter

1. Introduction

Anterior open bite (AOB) is a term used if there is localized absence of occlusion anteriorly when the remaining teeth are in occlusion; it is commonly one of the main symptoms of an overall dentofacial deformity. Diagnosis, treatment, and retention can be difficult because this malocclusion has numerous correlated etiologic factors. Clinically, it is grouped into 2 main categories: dental or acquired open-bites which have no distinguishing craniofacial malformations, and skeletal open bite with superimposed craniofacial dysplasia. [1]

The cause of an anterior open bite is multifactorial and can be attributed to a combination of skeletal, dental, and soft-tissue defects. Vertical malocclusion develops as a result of the interaction of many different etiologic factors including thumb and finger sucking, lip and tongue habits, airway obstruction, and true skeletal growth abnormalities. The etiologic factors play an important role in diagnosis. Heredity, unfavorable growth patterns and incorrect jaw postoure are the characteristics of skeletal AOB. Besides depending on where the thumb is placed, a number of different types of dental problems can develop. Malocclusions of the late mixed or permanent dentitions, caused by thumb sucking are not self-corrected and surely orthodontic treatment is necessary. Due to oral respiration, the mandible is postured inferiorly with the tongue protruded and resting against the oral floor. This postural alteration induces dental and skeletal modifications similar to those caused by thumb sucking. This may cause excessive eruption of the posterior teeth, leading to an increase in the vertical dimension of the face and result in development of AOB. Additionally, tongue habits cause an AOB or they develop secondarily to thumb sucking. In skeletal AOB the tongue habit acts as a secondary factor which helps to maintain or exacerbate the condition. Many orthodontists have had a discouraging experience of completing dental treatment, with what appeared to be good results, only to discover that the case had relapsed because the patient had a tongue thrust swallowing pattern. AOB is frequently observed in orthodontic practice. While 17.7% of children in the early to mixed dentition period present with an open bite of 1–12 mm [2], even after an improvement in orofacial dysfunctions [3], AOB is still diagnosed in 2.9% of adult Caucasian Americans [4]; it is an increasingly recognized major orthodontic problem. Patients with AOB malocclusion can be diagnosed clinically and cephalometrically; however, diagnosis should be viewed in the context of the skeletal and dental structure. Accurate classification of this malocclusion requires experience and training. Simple AOB during the exchange of primary to permanent dentition usually resolves without treatment. However, complex skeletal AOB that extend farther into the premolar and molar regions, and those that do not resolve by the end of the mixed dentition years may require orthodontic and/or surgical intervention. Most skeletal AOB cases are characterized by excessive vertical development of the posterior maxilla and usually have excessive eruption of posterior teeth accompanying AOB. [5] Treatment for AOB ranges from observation or simple habit control to complex surgical procedures. Successful identification of the etiology improves the chances of treatment success. Vertical growth is the last dimension to be completed, therefore treatment may appear to be successful at one point and fail later. Some treatment may be prolonged, if began early. When orthodontic or surgical intrusion of the overerupted maxillary teeth is performed, the mandible rotates closed at rest and in function, resulting in open-bite closure. [6] Different treatment modalities have been used for this purpose such as orthognathic surgery, conventional orthodontic appliances and combined methods. Orthodontic treatment options include functional appliances, and orthopedic devices. Intrusion of the overerupted molar teeth by traditional orthodontic methods is hardly possible in adult patients; there is therefore no real alternative to a combined orthodontic and surgical approach because the condition tends to recur after orthodontic treatment alone. In adult patients, combined approaches of surgery and orthodontic appliances make it possible to complete orthodontic treatment in a fast and predictable manner. [7]-[11] In the present chapter, advantages and disadvantages of current treatment protocols and corticotomy-facilitated compressive force procedure using orthodontic anchor plates applications are discussed in light of the current clinical literature.

2. Current clinical applications for treating severe AOB

2.1. Traditional orthodontic treatment options for AOB

Long-term skeletal and dental stability has been a concern because of the influence that the neuromusculature has on the repositioned jaws and the stability of teeth after vertical orthodontic mechanics required for closing open bites. Traditional treatment modalities include compensating orthodontics, functional appliances, and orthopedic devices. Orthodontic treatment involves extrusion of incisors or intrusion of molars. These therapies show relatively stable results for younger patients. In young patients, the vertical maxillary growth can be controlled with a high-pull headgear or a functional appliance with bite blocks. Once

excessive vertical development of the posterior maxilla has occurred, only two treatment options are available for the correction of an openbite. Elongation of the anterior teeth leaves
the skeletal component of the deformity unchanged. However, traditional techniques are
concluded to produce only relative intrusion of the molars and have a limited effect in providing sound anchorage. [12] The ideal period to begin open bite treatment is during the
mixed dentition; if the malocclusion is corrected during the deciduous dentition, it will recur because of continued growth changes. In the mixed dentition, the most important step in
correcting an open bite associated with abnormal habits is to eliminate the habits with be-
havior-modification techniques, accompanied by speech therapy; if necessary, a removable
functional appliance with a vertical crib can be used. It is important to present this treatment
to the child as an aid and not as a penalty. In about half of the patients, thumb sucking
ceases immediately, and the anterior open bite closes relatively quickly. After the habit is
eliminated, it is important to maintain the appliance for 3 to 6 months. However, when the
open bite is associated with skeletal features such as an increased mandibular plane angle,
anterior face height, and extruded posterior teeth, it is necessary to redirect maxillary
growth with molar intrusion, to rotate the mandible in an upward and forward direction.
[13] On the other hand, if the skeletal relationship is the primary cause of the AOB and control of the sucking habit is limited, the prognosis is poor. [14] The treatment of choice for this
problem is to reduce the vertical dimension by reducing the height of the posterior teeth.
The difficulty of managing anterior open-bite malocclusions is not only in obtaining the correct diagnosis, but also in treating a successful facial and dental result. The orthodontist's
challenge is to minimize molar extrusion during treatment to prevent downward and backward mandibular rotation. The early treatment strategy of skeletal AOB is based on inhibition of the vertical development or intrusion of the buccal dentoalveolar structures by
means of bite-blocks or extraoral appliances, thus producing upward and forward rotation
of the mandible into a more horizontal, rather than vertical growth direction. Early intercep-
tion offers psychological benefits and the potential for condylar growth. Nonsurgical options usually require longer treatment times and greater patient compliance. Although
attempts to limit the increase in vertical dimensions by at least 1 of the above approaches
were done by orthodontists, posterior bite-blocks proved to be effective in producing condylar growth and forward rotation of the mandible. To actively intrude the posterior teeth, active components in the form of magnets and springs have been suggested. [13]-[23]

The design of spring-loaded bite-blocks was first described by Woodside and Linder-Aron-
son. These blocks are activated from time to time, and they supply additional force in the
neuromuscular system, in addition to the forces of the masticatory muscles that are exerted
by the passive posterior bite-blocks. Because of its peculiar design, it was thought that the
same appliance could also act as a habit-breaking appliance. With this appliance, the patient
must apply active force to close his mouth, and this acts as a distraction device. By intruding
the posterior teeth, the mandible autorotates upward and forward. This form of treatment is
advantageous because it corrects the AOB and simultaneously reduces the total anterior facial height. The increase in muscle strength because of its oral dynamic effect ensures a stable result. A modified acrylic occlusal splint along with spring-loaded bite blocks have been
used to correct the skeletal AOB during the mixed dentition was shown to be efficient, but

its correct indication and control are of fundamental importance. Many approaches have been suggested to modify this early developmental pattern, but only posterior bite-blocks proved to be effective in producing condylar growth and forward rotation of the mandible. [14]-[23] To actively intrude the posterior teeth, Iscan et al., Akkaya and Haydar suggested the use of a spring-loaded bite-block. When adult patients are treated using classical orthodontic appliances, the duration of the treatments increase and risks such as root and marginal alveolar bone resorption, undesired movements of anchorage teeth, and relapse occur. Dental stability after vertical orthodontic mechanics is unpredictable and is prone to relapse. [24] Relapse is multifactorial and can involve skeletal and dentoalveolar components.

2.2. Orthognathic surgery techniques for AOB

Orthognathic surgery techniques for the treatment of AOB have been used for many years. The most frequently performed surgical procedures for AOB is correction via superior repositioning of the maxilla via LeFort I osteotomy, posterior segmental maxillary osteotomy, and vertical ramus osteotomy. Early attempts to close an AOB with mandibular procedures were mainly segmental [25], but were soon replaced by posterior impaction of the maxilla at LeFort I level as this was thought to be more stable. [26]-[28] If the mandible does not rotate into the correct position after the maxilla is impacted, 2-jaw surgery is required. The fear of surgery or general anesthesia and other factors may lead a significant proportion of patients to refuse surgery. Fewer than half of their patients who had sought orthodontic treatment for long-face problems accepted the recommended orthognathic surgery. Proffit et al., considered that a patient with a skeletal long-face problem who refused surgical correction was better left untreated. However, after initially successful correction of the vertical dimension by a combined treatment with a multibracket appliance and bimaxillary osteotomies, some of these patients with primary open bite may after treatment, experience a vertical relapse with a reduction in the overbite, or the reappearance of the anterior open bite. At post-treatment follow-up, the relapse rate ranged from 12% to roughly 30% depending on the type of treatment [29]-[34] In patients with severe AOB, secondary orthodontic therapy or repeated surgery may become necessary. The main indication for treatment of an AOB by posterior maxillary impaction is the presence of posterior maxillary vertical maxillary excess, which is common. About one third of patients who present with orthognathic concerns have vertical maxillary excess. It is also reported that about 60%of patients with it also have an openbite, or a tendency to an openbite. [35] It follows that many patients who are operated on to correct AOB may require maxillary surgery. Where the vertical and anterior–posterior position of the maxilla is within reasonable limits there is less of an indication to operate on the maxilla, except when it is thought to be the most stable technique to close an AOB. Although many studies have reported better stability with a maxillary procedure, the patients are heterogeneous and include those with appreciable vertical maxillary discrepancies. [36],[37] Few compare or report on cases where the maxilla was in a favourable position without a posterior vertical maxillary extension. The height of the mandibular ramus and the clinical state of the condyles are factors only recently emphasised as useful contributors to aiding the decision about the choice of procedure. [35]

Patients with a short mandibular ramus, normal condyles, no sign of ongoing resorption, and a well positioned maxilla would lend themselves to a mandibular sagittal split osteotomy (MSSO) alone as the procedure of choice. There have been few publications about mandibular surgery alone, with the few studies published including sample sizes of only 15–30. [38],[39] This may reflect the limited number of cases that are appropriate for such a procedure, or may reflect the blanket treatment selected by many, based on the heterogeneous case-mix previously analyzed, which universally suggests more stability with maxillary surgery. [40] Studies that describe or compare mandibular anticlockwise rotational movements alone do not clarify the technique of sagittal split osteotomy, and whether this was conventional or modified. In particular, with reference to the posterior extension of the cutinthe medial ramus, ensuring a split that allows part of the medial pterygoid to remain attached to the proximal segment and to stripping of the pterygomasseteric sling, medial pterygoid, and stylomandibular ligament from the distal segment. [35] These manoeuvres during a modified medial ramus osteotomy named as "short split technique" [26] reduce the risk that the medial pterygoid muscle may contribute to forces that encourage relapse when closing an AOB with the mandible. Other factors thought to contribute to relapse are the stretching of nonmuscular soft tissue and neuromuscular activity. Both factors are thought to adapt early postoperatively rather than cause relapse. Various studies have suggested that rigid fixation confers greater stability than other methods in the closure of AOB. [41] It has been suggested that rigid fixation using positional screws in the closure of an AOB may confer better surgical stability than semirigid mini-plates, and was therefore the preferred method used by the surgeons in this study. [36],[38],[41],[42]

Although maxillary osteotomy is done regularly with few complications, morbidity still exists and can be life threatening, especially if there is severe bleeding. In clinical practice, some patients who need closure of an AOB may also require an increased prominence of the chin. This would necessitate advancement genioplasty if the correction of the AOB was to be achieved by maxillary surgery only. Anticlockwise rotation of the mandible has the esthetic advantage of addressing this deficit, and avoids the risks and morbidity associated to advancement genioplasty as an additional procedure. Although there are few published reports, a growing numbers of surgeons are attempting and reporting MSSO technique to close AOB. [35],[38]-[40] Bimaxillary surgery, although advocated in the closure of AOB, may present a higher risk of morbidity than either maxillary or mandibular surgery alone. Published evidence has recognized the risks of relapse with this procedure [37],[43] and means that care must be taken in calculating the definite need for double jaw surgery to optimize the risk-to-benefit ratio for the patient.

This surgical procedure has not been well accepted because of rigid fixation, the need to use bone grafts and membranes, severe bleeding, longer duration of hospitalization, the risk of dental and periodontal problems that may occur when the bone segments are rapidly and excessively separated and increased risk of relapse. [44]

2.3. Titanium implants or bone anchors for AOB

AOB due to posterior maxillary dentoalveolar hyperplasia can be closed without orthognathic surgery. Osseointegrated implants serve as absolute anchorage for the intrusion of
over-erupted teeth; and, after tooth movement, can be used as restorative abutments. Patients who do not need prosthetic rehabilitation may benefit from a removable skeletal an-
choring device that can be placed outside the dentition. Absolute anchorage can only be
achieved if the anchorage devices are fixed in bone. Such devices include miniplates, miniscrews, palatal implants, onplants and dental implants. Anchorage control is a prerequisite
for the success of orthodontic treatment. Loss of dental anchorage during orthodontic treatment leads to uncontrolled occlusion results. Recent clinical studies regarding AOB suggesting the use of skeletal anchors with fixed Edgewise appliances, demonstrated that
incorporation of skeletal anchors was an excellent alternative to traditional orthodontic
treatment methods and may provide a significant amount of maxillary and/or mandibular
molar intrusion for AOB. The pure titanium miniplates that are well-known in maxillofacial
trauma and orthognathic surgery comply with these criteria.[11],[45]-[52] Several studies
have examined the effects of miniplates as anchors for orthodontic distal and intrusive
movements. [11],[12],[53]-[57] Miniplates placed outside the maxillary and mandibular dentition functioned as onplants, and the screws functioned as implants, making rigid anchorage possible. Rigid anchorage results from osseointegration of both anchor plates and
screws. Although there have been some promising casereports, there are few studies on the
posttreatment complications of miniplates used for orthodontic anchorage. Umemori et al.,
Sherwood et al. and Akay et al. reported that the miniplates in their studies were quite stable. However, some patients developed chronic infections related to the miniplates. Nowadays, for upper or lower molar intrusion, orthodontic implants, miniscrews and modified
titanium miniplates are used and recommended by different investigators. In a study by
Xun et al. on 12 patients with open bite malocclusions, upper and lower molars were intruded 1.8 mm and 1.2 mm, respectively, in a mean of 6.8 months with the use of micro-screws
as anchors. Several reports document that screw-type implants have been successful anchor-
ing units in general. [46],[56]-[59] Miyawaki et al. found that the 1-year success rate of
screws with 1.0-mm diameter was significantly less than that of other screws with 1.5-mm or
2.3-mm diameter or than that of miniplates. When compared with mini or micro-screws, titanium anchor plates hold the advantage of functioning as sound anchorage units against
increased force levels. [11],[12],[51]-[53],[55]-[61] Furthermore, a high-mandibular plane angle was found to be a potential risk factor for the failure of screw-type implant anchors and
the use of miniplates in patients with high mandibular plane angles were suggested when
micro-screws were risky to insert.[56] In a clinical study Akay et al. treated adults with
AOB, using titanium screws of 2.3 mm diameter and 7, 9, 13 mm lengths and their results
correlated with recent studies by Sherwood et al., Chung et al., De Clerck et al., Miyawaki et
al., Erverdi et al., Choi et al., and Erverdi et al. concluding that miniplates placed at zygomatic butresses and buccal bone above the roots of premolars remained stable following application of intrusive forces. In this study, no signs of mobility of titanium screws placed in
the palatal bone were observed.

Sherwood et al. and Erverdi et al. supported orthodontic forces by implanting titanium miniplates at the lower face of the zygomatic process of maxilla aiming to correct skelatal AOB. Sherwood et al.2002 demonstrated a mean upper molar intrusion of 1.99 mm with intrusive forces continued for 5.5 months in four patients whereas Erverdi et al.2004 reported a mean maxillary molar intrusion of 2.6 mm in 10 patients after a mean of 5.1 months. Yao et al.2005, used a combination of a buccal miniplate and palatal miniscrew in 18 patients and buccal and palatal miniscrews in 4 patients who had overerupted maxillary molars. They reported that the mean intrusion of maxillary first molars was 3 to 4 mm in a mean of 7.6 months.Titanium miniplates implanted in the zygomatic buttress area can serve as absolute anchorage for maxillary molar intrusion. Recent studies suggesting the use skeletal anchors with fixed Edgewise appliances demonstrated that incorporation of skeletal anchors was an excellent alternative to traditional methods and may provide a significant amount of maxillary and/or mandibular molar intrusion. [12],[47],[48],[50]-[53],[61]-[63]

Titanium miniplates are strongly recommended for temporary skeletal anchorage. Both the placement and the removal of the plates are minimally invasive procedures with only slight discomfort to the patient and with no serious side effects. The dense cortical bone of the zygomatic buttress area is an ideal miniplate anchorage site for maxillary molar intrusion. Development of miniature bone anchors have made this clinically feasible and practical. In the literature, a wide range of intrusion forces between 100 and 900 g was suggested for intrusion of maxillary molars, in nongrowing individuals. [45],[47],[50],[52],[64],[65] However, the optimal force to be applied following corticotomy is not clear.[11] Park et al. used 200-300 g of force for intrusion of maxillary posterior teeth with 3 roots, without a corticotomy procedure. After a buccal and palatal corticotomy Akay et al. applied an intrusion force of 200-300 g on each molar and two premolars, considering that with force level less than 200 g, intrusion may be delayed and alveolar bone may heal prematurely. On the other hand, a force level greater than 300 g may stimulate root resorption. It has been suggested that subapical corticotomy procedure decreases the risk of root resoption because the bone blocks are moved with the teeth. [9],[11],[52],[66],[67]

2.4. Corticotomy assisted maxillary impaction with bone anchor miniplates

Patients with skeletal AOB are considered the most difficult to manage because the condition tends to recur after treatment, particularly after single-jaw osteotomy. [32],[68] Patients would almost certainly prefer a less invasive surgical procedure with little or no risk and less discomfort. Additionally, a slow change in the facial appearance may be more acceptable for some patients than a sudden one. Besides local rather than general anesthesia, a decreased operation time, and a shorter duration of hospitalization can reduce costs.[69] A combination of subapical corticotomy and orthodontic treatment supported with bone anchors may be an alternative method for skeletal AOB correction in adult patients who would like to consider a rather rapid treatment option. Recently, surgically assisted orthodontic treatment for severe AOB has been described that has the advantages of corticotomy facilitated orthodontic treatment using orthodontic-skeletal anchorage miniplates. Combined approaches of surgery and orthodontic appliances make it possible to complete orthodontic treatment in a rapid and predictable manner. Anchor plate or implant appliances allow reliable and expedient orthodontic treatment with minimal orthodontic anchorage loss. It has been suggested that corticotomy procedure decreases the risk of root resoption because the bone blocks are moved with the teeth; this compression osteogenesisis osteoplasty technique is based on the distraction osteogenesis phenomenon. [7]-[11],[57],[66],[71],[72]

Chung et al.used an orthodontic anchor plate system in his clinical study. According to the study, the teeth were moved in a block of bone that was connected to other teeth and anchored via low-density medullary bone and the block was repositioned on an outpatient basis using anchor plates and orthodontic elastics under local anaesthesia. Although this method is also indicated for open-bite patients without anterior–posterior dentofacial problems, the author's new surgical approach decreases the time required for treatment by allowing rapid movement of a block of teeth and bone. It is widely accepted that the utilization of corticotomy before orthodontic treatment allows positively accelerated tooth movement thereby shortening active treatment time with less risk of root resoption and more stable results as well. [9],[11],[52],[66],[67] Akay et al. recently described the efficacy of this technique in combination with a buccal and palatal corticotomy using a bone anchor miniplate system. After one-step corticotomy, the posterior teeth were moved in a block of bone that was connected to other teeth and anchored via low density medullary bone (Figs. 1a-d).

Although corticotomy has become an alternative technique for maxillofacial surgeons, there is no consensus in the literature regarding corticotomy assisted bone anchors application used in maxillary impaction, type of bone anchors used, effects of the new technique on the TMJ, teeth or skeletal structures, the cause and amount of relapse and whether or not overcorrection is necessary. Clinical results of Akay et al. showed that this operation can be performed succesfully under local anesthesia without sedation in cooperative patients.

There are some controversies regarding the type of corticotomy before bone anchor miniplates are inserted.

Subapical corticotomy technique used by Akay et al.: Under local anesthesia the corticotomies are performed prior to implantation of skeletal anchors. The vertical cuts begin 2 to 3 mm above the alveolar crest and extend 5 to 6 mm beyond the tooth apicies. The vertical cuts are made within the compact bone barely reaching the medullary bone on the mesial side of the most anterior tooth and on the distal side of the most posterior tooth to be intruded. A horizontal cut is then made 4 to 5 mm above the apices of the relevant teeth and connected to the 2 vertical cuts. The resection gap is 3 to 4 mm wide to facilitate the intrusion. These cuts are made on both the buccal and palatal sides so that the block of bone is retained only by the medullary bone.

For intrusion of molars, zygoma anchors with three holes (Surgi-Tec, Brugge, Belgium) are adjusted to fit the contour of the bone of each zygomatic process of the maxilla using a plate shaping kit and fixed by three 2.3 mm wide and 7 to 9 mm length miniscrews (Surgi-Tec, Brugge, Belgium). In order to intrude premolars, miniplates with two holes (Surgi-Tec, Brugge, Belgium) are attached 6-7 mm above the roots of relevant teeth and are stabilized by titanium screws (2.3 mm in diameter and 5-7 mm in length (Surgi-Tec, Brugge, Belgium).To prevent any possible buccal tipping of posterior treeth during intrusion, two titanium screws (2.3 mm in diameter and 13 mm in length, Surgi-Tec, Brugge, Belgium) are implanted in the palatal region between the molars and between the premolars bilaterally, these aided as anchors for applying additional palatal force vectors (Figs. 2-4).

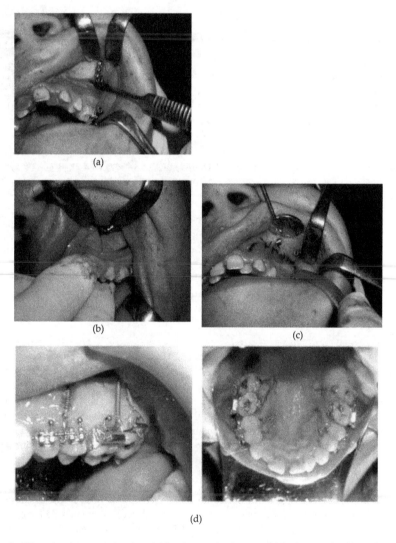

(a)

(b)   (c)

(d)

Figure 1. a) Operative photograph showing miniplate bone anchor insertion. (b) The horizontal and vertical corticotomy on the buccal surface. (c) Postoperative clinical appearance showing bone anchor position (d) Postoperative clinical photograph showing intrusive force application (buccal view left, palatal right).

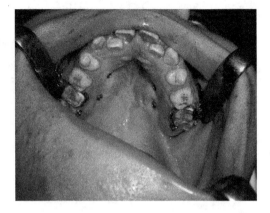

Figure 2. Clinical appearence of screws implanted in the palatal region between the molars and between the premolars bilaterally.

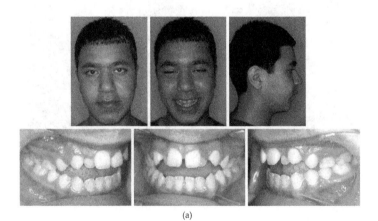

(a)

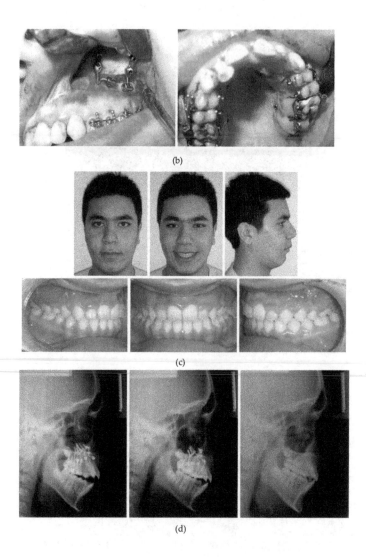

(b)

(c)

(d)

Figure 3. a. Clinical appearence of Case 1 and preoperative intraoral photographs showing severe anterior open bite. b. Intraoperative photograph showing buccal and palatal corticotomy and buccal miniplates and palatal screws insertion. c. Postoperative facial photographs and occlusion after completion of orthodontic treatment. d. Cephalometric views preoperatively, during molar intrusion and after completion of orthodontic treatment.

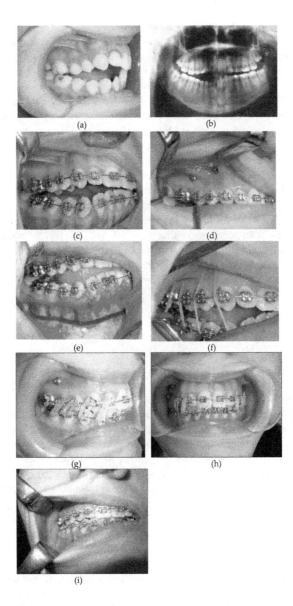

Figure 4. a. Clinical appearance of case 2 and (b) preoperative ortopantomograph showing severe open bite. c. Ortho-dontic preparation and (d) screw applications on the maxilllary posterior buccal cortex. e. The corticotomy on the mandibular buccal surface and (f) compression force activated using elastics. g. Lateral and (h) anterior clinical photo-graphs during dentoalveolar osteogenesis. i. Postoperative photograph showing occlusion after completion of ortho-dontic treatment.

According to clinical study by Kanno et al., the two-stage segmental corticotomy technique may be performed under local anaesthesia with intravenous sedation and avoiding the need for conventional orthognathic surgery. Although complex double-jaw surgery is considered a relatively routine intervention for patients with severe anterior open bite, bimaxillary surgery under general anaesthesia may lead to complications necessitating intense postoperative care. [32],[68],[73] None of the postoperative complications, including root resorption, loss of tooth vitality, periodontal problems, pocket formation and segmental malunion, were observed that have been associated with less invasive surgical treatments. [10],[11],[70],[71] Although AOB may be improved by concurrent counterclockwise rotation of the mandible and molar intrusion with skeletal anchor plates, the molar intrusion is limited, the new combined technique allows postoperative adjustment of the bone/teeth segments to the ideal position using a gradual compressive force over a shortened treatment period. [10],[11],[57] An orthodontist performed post-surgical management on an out-patient basis. Reliable control of the corticotomy-facilitated teeth/bone segments has been reported in studies on bone biology and remodelling with compressive induction. [10],[11],[70],[71] According to these authors, no postoperative relapse and complications, such as infectios, dentoalveolar fractures, TMJ symptoms, dental or periodontal problems, loss of tooth vitality, segmental malunion, loss of anchorage and fracture of miniplates and screws were observed during or after corticotomy surgery.

3. Conclusion

AOB is a common problem in orthognathic practice that causes functional and esthetic handicaps on affected patients and it is frequently discussed in orthodontics. Its management varies and it is one of the most challenging disorders to treat. The orthodontic and surgical approach to the treatment of skeletal AOB is still debated, and the results are still controversial. Diagnosis, treatment, and retention can be difficult because this malocclusion has numerous correlated etiologic factors. The earlier this malocclusion is corrected, the better the prognosis will be, especially when the problem is skeletal. Treatment is usually not necessary until permanent teeth erupt (approximately at the age of 6 year). There are different treatment modalities for AOB in the literature. However, many surgeons find it difficult to decide which technique offers better results, and are also uncertain about the factors which might influence their techniques of choice. Many adult patients with AOB are significantly compromised, requiring a multidisciplinary approach to treatment. It is very important to consider surgical and dental concerns during AOB treatment planning. The relapse rate is high with all the techniques in current use. The cause of relapse is multifactorial and one of the main factors is the type of osteotomy used. Corticotomy-facilitated bone anchor applications for treating AOB has become increasingly popular as an alternative to many conventional orthognathic surgical procedures. For patients with mild to severe abnormalities of the AOB, this combined technique has increased the number of treatment alternatives. Although long-term follow-up of occlusion stability is required, the recent evidence suggest that a corticotomy-facilitated compressive force procedure using orthodontic anchor plates is an effective means of treating patients with severe AOB, however further multicenter studies with a larger population are necessary to precisely evaluate postoperative relapse, other clinical complications and skeletal and dental changes in the long term. Further studies with different designs of titanium miniplates for orthodontic anchorage might be helpful in identifying factors for decreasing the incidence of complications. Improvement of the technique and devices used, with an adjusted protocol, could lead to a reduction in the number of complications.

Acknowledgment

I thank Professor Dr. Aynur Aras, for her orthodontic contributions to the chapter.

Author details

Mehmet Cemal Akay

Ege University, Faculty of Dentistry, Department of Oral and Maxillofacial Surgery, Izmir, Turkey

References

[1] Subtelny, J.D. & Sakuda M., (1964) Open-bite: diagnosis and treatment. *AmJ Orthod* Vol.50, pp:337-358

[2] Tausche, E., Luck O., Harzer W.,(2004) Prevalence of malocclusions in the early mixed dentition and orthodontic treatment need. Eur J Orthod Vol.26, No:3,pp: 237-244

[3] Ermel, T., Hoffmann J.& Alfter G., et al. (1999) Long-term stability of treatment results after upper jaw segmented osteotomy according to Schuchardt for correction of anterior open bite. *J Orofac Orthop Vol.*60, No:4, pp:236-245

[4] Proffit, W.R., Fields H.W. Jr.& Moray L.J., (1998) Prevalence of malocclusion and orthodontic treatment need in the United States: estimates from the NHANES III survey. *Int J Adult Orthodon Orthognath Surg*Vol.13, No:2, pp:97-106

[5] Schudy, F.F.(1965). The rotation of the mandible resulting from growth: itsimplications in orthodontic treatment. *Angle Orthod*Vol.35, pp:36-50

[6] Bell, W.H. & Proffit W.R.,(1980) Open bite. In: Bell WH, Proffit WR, White RP.eds. Surgical Correction of Dentofacial Deformities. Philadelphia, PA:Saunders, pp: 1058-1209

[7]   Kole, H., (1959) Surgical operations on the alveolar ridge to correct occlusal abnormalities. *Oral Surg Oral Med Oral Pathol* Vol.12, pp: 515–529

[8]   Kerdvongbundit, V., (1990) Corticotomy—facilitated orthodontics. *J Dent Assoc*Thai Vol.40, 284–291

[9]   Hwang, H.S.&Lee K.H., (2001) Intrusion of overerupted molars by corticotomy and magnets. *Am J Orthod Dentofacial Orthop*Vol.120, pp:209-216

[10] Kanno, T., Mitsugi1 M.&FurukiY., et al., (2007)Corticotomy and compression osteogenesis in the posterior maxilla for treating severe anterior open bite.*Int J Oral Maxillofac Surg*Vol. 36, pp: 354–357

[11] Akay, M.C., Aras A. & Günbay T., et al., (2010) Enhanced Effect of Combined Treatment with Corticotomy and Skeletal Anchorage in Open-bite Correction. J Oral Maxillofac Surg, Vol.67.No.3, pp: 563-569

[12] Sherwood, K.H., Burch J.G., Thompson W.J.,(2002) Closing anterior open bites by intruding molars with titanium miniplate anchorage. *Am J Orthod Dentofacial Orthop* Vol.122, pp:593-600

[13] Altuna, G.&WoodsideD.G., (1985) Response of the midface to treatment with increased vertical occlusal forces. *Angle Orthod* Vol.55,pp:251-263

[14] Cozza, P., Baccetti T.& Franchi L., et al., (2005) Sucking habits and facial hyper divergency as risk factors for anterior openbite in the mixed dentition. *Am J Orthod Dentofacial Orthop*Vol.128, pp:517-519

[15] Dellinger, E.L.)1986)A clinical assessment of the active vertical corrector, a nonsurgical alternative for skeletal open bite treatment. *Am J Orthod*Vol.89, pp:428-436

[16] Woods, M.G.&Nanda R.S., (1988)Intrusion of Posterior Teeth with Magnets. *The Angle Orthodontis*, Vol. 58, No:2, pp: 136-150

[17] Kalra, V.&Burstone C.J., (1989) Effects of a fixed magnetic appliance on the dentofacial complex. *Am J Orthod Dentofacial Orthop*Vol.95, pp:467-478

[18] Kiliaridis, S., Egermark I.&Thilander B., (1990) Anterior open bite treatment with magnets. *Eur J Orthod*Vol.12, pp:447-457

[19] Barbre, R.E.&Sinclair P.M.,(1991); A cephalometric evaluation of anterior open bite correction with the magnetic active vertical corrector.*Angle Orthod*Vol.61,pp:93-102.

[20] Akkaya,S.&Haydar S., (1996) Post-retention results of spring-loaded posteriorbite-block therapy. *Aust Orthod J*,Vol.14, pp:179-183

[21] Kuster, R &Ingervall B.,(1992) The effect of treatment of skeletal open bite with two types of bite-blocks. *Eur J Orthod*Vol.14, pp:489-499

[22] Iscan, H.N., Akkaya S.&Koralp E., (1992) The effects of the spring-loaded posterior bite- block on the maxillofacial morphology. *Eur J Orthod* Vol.14, pp:54-60

[23] Iscan, H.N.& Sarisoy L.,(1997)Comparison of the effects of passive posterior bite-blocks with different construction bites on the craniofacial and dentoalveolar structures. *Am J Orthod Dentofacial Orthop* Vol.112, pp:171-178

[24] Denison, T.F.,KokichV.G.&ShapiroP.A., (1989) Stability of maxillary surgery in open bite Versus non-open bite malocclusions. *Angle Orthod* Vol.59, pp:5–10

[25] Kloosterman,J., (1985) Koele's osteotomy: A follow-up study. *J MaxillofacSurg* Vol. 13:59–63.

[26] Epker, B.N.&Fish L. (1977) Surgical-orthodontic correction of open-bite deformity. *Am JOrthod*Vol.;71, pp:278–299

[27] Swinnen, K., Politis C. & Willems G., et al.,(2001) Skeletal and dento-alveolar stability after surgical-orthodontic treatment of anterior open bite: a retrospective study. *Eur JOrthod*Vol.23, pp:547-557

[28] Schmidt L.P. & Sailer H., (1991) Long-term results of surgical-orthodontic treatment of open bite deformity by a LeFort-I osteotomy. *Swiss Dent* Vol.27, No:29,pp:31–32

[29] Epker, B.N.(1981) Superior surgical repositioning of the maxilla: long term results.*J Max-Fac Surg*Vol.9, pp: 237-246

[30] Lo, F. & Shapiro P., (1998) Effect of presurgical incisor extrusionon stability of anterior open bite malocclusion treated with orthognathic surgery. *Int JAdult Orthod Orthognath Surg*Vol.13, pp:23–34

[31] Espeland, L., Dowling P.A. & Mobarak .KA., et al., (2008) Three-year stability of open-bite correction by 1-piece maxillary osteotomy. *Am J Orthod Dentofacial Orthop* Vol.134, No:1,pp:60-66

[32] Fischer, K., Von Konow L. & Brattstrom V. (2000)Open bite: stability after bimaxillary surgery—2-year treatment outcomes in58 patients. *Eur J Orthod*Vol. 22, pp:711–718

[33] Hoppenreijs, T.J., van der Linden F.P. & Freihofer H.P., et al., (1996) Occlusal and functional conditions after surgical correction of anterior open bite deformities. *Int J Adult Orthodon Orthognath Surg*Vol.11, No:1,pp:29-39

[34] Hoppenreijs, T.J., Freihofer H.P. & Stoelinga P.J., et al., (1997) Skeletal and dento-alveolar stability of LeFort I intrusion osteotomies and bimaxillary osteotomies in anterior open bite deformities. A retrospective three-centre study. *Int J Oral Maxillofac Surg* Vol.26, pp:161-175

[35] Reyneke, J.P. & Ferretti C., (2007) Anterior openbite correction by LeFort I or bilateral sagittal split osteotomy. *Oral Maxillofac Surg Clin North Am* Vol.19, pp:321–328

[36] Hoppenreijs, T.J., Freihofer H.P. & Stoelinga P.J., et al., (2001) Stability of Orthodontic Maxillofacial surgical treatment of anterior openbite deformities. Ned Tijdschr Tandheelkd Vol.108,pp:173–178

[37] Proffit, W.R., Bailey L.J.& Phillips C, Turvey TA.(2000) Long-term stability of surgical open bite correction by LeFort I osteotomy. *Angle Orthod*Vol.70, pp:112-7

[38] Oliveira, JA & Bloomquist, D.S. (1997)The stability of the use of bilateral sagittal split Osteotomy in the closure of anterior openbite. *Int J Adult Orthodon Orthognath Surg*Vol.12, pp:101–108

[39] Reitzik, M., Barer P.G. & Wainwright W.M., et al., (1990); The surgical treatment of skeletal anterior open-bite deformities with rigid internal fixation in the mandible. *Am J Orthod Dentofacial Orthop* Vol.97, No:1, pp:52-57

[40] Bisase, B., Johnson P. & Stacey M., (2010) Closure of the anterior openbite using mandibular Sagittal split osteotomy. *British J Oral Maxillofac Surg* Vol.48, pp:352–355

[41] Blomqvist, J.E., Ahlborg G. & Isaksson S., et al., (1997)A comparison of skeletal stability after Mandibular advancement and use of two rigid internal fixation techniques. *J Oral Maxillofac Surg.*Vol.55, pp:568–575

[42] Forssell, K., Turwey T.A. & Philips C., et al., (1992)Superior repositioning ofthe maxilla combined with mandibular advancement: mandibular" RiF improves , stability. *Am J Orthod Dentofac Orthop* Vol.102, pp:-342-350

[43] Proffit, W.R., Turvey T.A. & Phillips C., (2007) The hierarchy of stability and predictability in orthognathic surgery with rigid fixation: an update and extension. *Head Face Med*Vol.30, No:3, pp:21

[44] Martin, D.L.,(1998) Transverse stability of multi-segmented Le Fort I expansion procedures (Master's thesis). Dallas: Baylor College of Dentistry

[45] Park, H.S., Kwon T.G. & Jang B.K., et al.,(2004) Treatment of open bite with microscrew implant anchorage. *Am J Orthod Dentofacial Orthop*Vol.126, pp:627-635

[46] Park, H.S., Lee S.K. & Kwon O.W., (2005) Group distal movement of teeth using microscrew implant anchorage. *Am J Orthod Dentofacial Orthop*Vol.75, pp:602-609

[47] Park, H.S., Kwon O.W. & Sung J.H. (2006) Nonextraction treatment of an open bite with micro screw implant anchorage. *Am J Orthod Dentofacial Orthop*Vol.130,pp: 391-402

[48] Yao, C.C., Wu C.B., Wu H.Y., et al., (2005) Maxillary molar intrusion with fixed appliances and mini-implant anchorage studied in three dimensions. *Angle Orthod*Vol.75, pp :754-760

[49] Kuroda, S., Sakai Y. & Tamamura N., et al.,(2007) Treatment of severe anterior open bite with skeletal anchorage in adults: Comparison with orthognathic surgery outcomes. *Am J Orthod Dentofacial Orthop*Vol.132, pp:599-605

[50] Xun, C., Zeng X., & Wang X.,(2007) Microscrew Anchorage in skeletal anterior openbite treatment. *Angle Orthod* Vol. 77,pp:47-56

[51] Erverdi, N., Keles A. & Nanda R., (2004) The use of skeletal anchorage in open bite treatment: a cephalometric evaluation. *Angle Orthod*Vol.74, pp:381-390

[52] Erverdi, N., Usumez S. & Solak A. (2006) New generation open-bite treatment with zygomatic anchorage. *Angle Orthod*Vol.76, pp:519-526

[53] Umemori, M., Sugawara J. & Mitani H, et al., (1999) Skeletal anchorage system for open-bite correction. *Am J Orthod Dentofacial Orthop*Vol.15, pp:166–174

[54] Daimaruya, T., Nagasaka H. & Umemori M., et al., (2001) The influences of molar intrusion on the inferior alveolar neurovascular bundle and root using the skeletal anchorage system in dogs. *Angle Orthod*Vol.71,pp:60-70

[55] De Clerck, H., Geerinckx V. & Siciliano S., (2002) The zygoma anchorage system. *J Clin Orthod*Vol.36,pp:455-459

[56] Miyawaki, S., Koyama I. & Inoue M., et al., (2003) Factors associated with the stability of titanium screws placed in the posterior region for orthodontic anchorage. *Am J Orthod Dentofacial Orthop*Vol.124, pp:373–378

[57] Sugawara, J., Baik U.B. & Umemori M., et al., (2002) Treatment and post-treatment Dentoalveolar changes following intrusion of mandibular molars with application of a skeletal anchorage system (SAS) for open bite correction. *Int J Adult Orthod Orthognath Surg*Vol.17, pp:243-245

[58] Liou, E.J., Pai B.C. & Lin J.C., (2004) Do miniscrews remain stationary under orthodontic forces? *Am J Orthod Dentofacial Orthop*Vol.126,pp:42-47

[59] Chen, C.H., Chang C.S. & Hsieh C.H., et al.,(2006) The use of microimplants in orthodontic anchorage. *J Oral Maxillofac Surg*Vol.64,pp:1209-1213

[60] Choi, B.H., Zhu S.J. & Kim Y.H. (2005) A clinical evaluation of titanium miniplates as anchors for orthodontic treatment. *Am J Orthod Dentofacial Orthop*Vol.128, pp:382-384

[61] Chung, K.R., Kım Y.S. & Linton J.L., et al., (2002) The miniplate with tube for skeletal anchorage. *J Clin Orthod*Vol.36, pp::407-412

[62] Costa, A., Raffini M., & Melsen B., (1998) Miniscrews as orthodontic anchorage:a preliminary report. *Int J Adult Orthod Orthognath Surg Vol.*13,pp:201-209

[63] Seres, L. & Kocsis A., (2009) Open-bite closure by intruding maxillary molars with skeletalanchorage. In: Bell W, Guerrero C. eds. Distraction Osteogenesis of the Facial Skeleton. Hamilton, Ontario, Canada: BCDecker, pp:215-220

[64] Park, Y.C., Lee S.Y & Kim D.H., et al., (2003) Intrusion of posterior teeth using miniscrew implants. *Am J Orthod Dentofacial Orthop*Vol.123, pp:690-694

[65] Carano, A., Siciliani G. & Bowman S.J. (2005) Treatment of skeletal open bite witha device forrapid molar intrusion. *Angle Orthod Vol.*75, pp:736-746

[66] Suya H. Corticotomy in orthodontics. In:Hösl E, Baldauf A, editors. Mechanical and biological basis in orthodontic therapy. Heidelberg: Hüthig, 1991, p.207-226

[67] Mostafa, Y.A., Tawfik K.M., El-Mangoury N.H., (1985) Surgical-orthodontic treat-
      ment for overerupted maxillary molars. *J Clin Orthod*Vol.19, pp:350-351

[68] Burford, D. & Noar J.H., (2003) The causes, diagnosis and treatment of anterior open
      bite. *Dent Update Vol. 30*, pp: 235–241

[69] Proffit, W.R., White R.P. & Sarver D.M.,(2003)Long face problems. In: Proffit WR,
      White RP, Sarver DM, eds. Contemporary Treatment of Dentofacial Deformity. St
      Louis, MO:Mosby, pp:464-506

[70] Sen, C., Kocaoglu M. & Eralp L., et al., (2004) Bifocal compression-distraction in the
      acute treatment of grade IIIopen tibia fractures with bone and soft tissue loss: a re-
      port of24 cases.*J Orthop Trauma*Vol. 18, pp: 150–157

[71] Kawakami, T., Nishimoto M. & Matsuda Y., et al., (1996) Histological suture changes
      following retraction of the maxillary anterior bone segment after corticotomy. *Endod
      Dent Traumatol* Vol.12, pp:38–43

[72] Chung, K.R., Oh M.Y. & Ko S.J. (2001) Corticotomy-assisted orthodontics. *J Clin Or-
      thod* Vol.35, pp: 331–339

[73] Panula, K., Keski-Nisula L., Keski-Nisula K., et al., (2002) Costs of surgical-orthodon-
      tic treatment in community hospital care: an analysis of the different phases of treat-
      ment. *Int J Adult Orthod Orthognath Surg*Vol.17,pp:297-306

Temporomandibular Joint Disorders and Facial Pain

Chapter 8

Diagnosis and Management of Temporomandibular Disorders

Fina Navi, Mohammad Hosein Kalantar Motamedi,
Koroush Taheri Talesh, Esshagh Lasemi and
Zahra Nematollahi

Additional information is available at the end of the chapter

1. Introduction

Temporomandibular disorder (TMD) is one of the most common disorders in the maxillofacial region which usually presents with pain, unusual sounds, discomfort in chewing and locking of the jaw. TMD patients comprise a considerable proportion of patients seeking treatment; early diagnosis is important because it is proven that acute TMD responds well to treatment in contrast to chronic TMD. True diagnosis and treatment of TMD can be difficult, as these patients often suffer from some other disorder at the same time. In these cases, a successful treatment is due to true diagnosis of all initiating factors, predisposing and perpetuating factors and treatment of other established disorders. An important point is the close relation of intrajoint disorders to disorders of masticatory muscles. Today, it has been proven that disorder of masticatory muscles can lead to TMD. The opposite of this, is also true. Correct diagnosis is essential. The diagnostic steps and differential diagnosis of TMD and the treatment protocols from supportive treatment, splint therapy and physiotherapy to temporomandibular joint (TMJ) surgeries are explained herein. We hope this chapter can help better understand TMJ disorders, diagnosis and recognition of the signs and symptoms of disorders of the temporomandibular and masticatory system.

2. Temporomandibular disorder (TMD)

TMD is a general term including clinical problems which affect masticatory muscles, TMJ and adjacent structures. TMD is the most common non-dental pain in the maxillofacial region. The most common sign of TMD is pain in masticatory muscles, or preauricular region and on the TMJ which becomes severe when chewing or upon other mandibular movements. TMD patients have limitation and asymmetry in mandibular movements. They often have clicking, popping, grating and crepitus. Patients may complain from headache, earache and pain in the mandibulofacial region. Masticatory muscle hypertrophy and an unusual facet of occlusal surfaces of the dentition due to excessive mandibular movements such as bruxism or grinding may be present. Management of TMJ disorders usually includes finding the cause or etiology. Parafunction and trauma are common causes of TMD. Stress and mental problems are secondary aggravating factors. [1,2]

2.1. History

After initial studies in 1934, Costen proposed that patients suffering from auricular pain, pressure and fullness in the ear and swallowing problems (Costen syndrome) improve by occlusion correction. In the 1960s, the quality of clinical examinations and scientific studies improved; the importance of occlusion in TMD etiology in 1970 was studied. Methods including tomography, arthrography, computed tomography (CT) scan and magnetic resonance imaging (MRI) lead to improvements in examination of intracapsular structures. Today the information in this field show that patients with orofacial pains may suffer from disorders such as systemic, neuromuscular, vascular, and mental or a combination of disorders associated with TMD; some headway in pain mechanism, neurology, physiology and neuoropharmacology have been made. Different studies demonstrated that TMD treatment has changed based on the diagnosis of the etiology and stage of the disorder. [1,2]

2.2. TMJ anatomy

Temporomandibular joint is the junction site of the mandibular condyle to skull base or glenoid fossa of the temporal bone. A disc separates the two bones. The part of the disc which is in contact with mandibular condyle bone consists of fibrous connective tissue without any nerve or vessel. This joint is a compound one. The disc is divided into three parts, in sagittal view: anterior, posterior and middle. The middle zone is the thinnest part. The disc becomes thicker in the anterior and posterior parts. In coronal view, the medial part of the disc is thicker than the lateral part (Fig. 1). [1]

Disc shape is determined by condyle morphology and mandibular fossa. The disc may become displaced or destroyed via degenerative forces. In the posterior part, the disc is attached to a loose connective tissue of nerve and vessels named retrodiscal tissue. In the superior posterior part, it is attached to a connective tissue full of elastic bands named superior retrodiscal layer or bilaminary zone. This tissue connects the disc to the tympanic bone posteriorly. Below this, there is the inferior retrodiscal layer which connects the inferior border of the posterior edge of the disc to the posterior part of condyle joint surface. Inferior disc layer and superior retrodiscal tissue are made of collagen and elastic fibers, respectively. Anteriorly to the disc, superior and inferior adhesions of it connect to the capsular ligament. Both of these adhesions are made of collagen fibers. Between the capsular ligaments, the disc is adherent to fibers of the superior lateral pterygoid muscle. The disc adheres to the capsular ligament, not only anteroposterior-

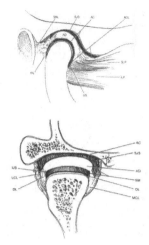

Figure 1. TMJ in sagittal and coronal views.

ly, but also mediolaterally. The joint is divided into two separate and distinct spaces. The superior space is located between the glenoid fossa and superior part of the disc; the inferior disc space lies between the disc and condyle. Internal surfaces of superior and inferior spaces are lined with special endothelial cells which secrete synovial fluid. This fluid has two functions: 1-Molecular transport and metabolism and 2-Lubrication of joint surfaces; the fluid is secreted on the joint surfaces under pressure and results in friction reduction. During function, forces entering to the joint surfaces lead to movement of this fluid into intrajoint tissues. In coronal view, the condyle has a medial and lateral pole; the medial pole is thicker than the lateral one. The TMJ is supported by three major and two minor ligaments. [1,2]

Major ligaments are:

1. Collateral ligaments

2. Capsular ligament

3. Temporomandibular ligament

Minor ligaments are:

1. Sphenomandibular ligament

2. Stylomandibular ligament

2.3. TMD etiology

TMD is considered as a multifactorial disorder and there is no special or individual cause for it. There are factors which can damage the balance in TMJ and the masticatory system. Bone deformations, soft tissue metaplasia of TMJ and muscle activity reduction are often adaptive responses to changes. Hyperactivity of masticatory muscles resulting from parafunctional habits can lead to adaptive responses in dynamic balance because of hyperactivity and high load in the long term. Excessive changes in any of the above functions can lead to disability to adapt leading to TMJ disorders. For example, external trauma to any part results in injuries and disorders in normal joint function. Moreover, anatomic, systemic, pathophysiological and emotional causes can make the disorder more severe. [1,2]

2.3.1. Trauma

Nowadays, trauma is believed to be the initial cause of TMD. In fact, excessive trauma because of parafunctional forces can damage the masticatory system. These damages may result in joint injuries and pain in eating, smiling, yawing or excessive opening of the mouth. External trauma such as a punch, sport activities and injuries because of dental practice can lead to TMD. An important type of trauma is parafunctional trauma. Postural habits such as head forwarding or holding the phone handset place pressure on joints and muscles which result in musculoskeletal pains such as headaches in TMD patients. Additional habits and movements such as clenching, bruxism, attrition, lip biting and abnormal posture of the jaws common in society may lead to TMD. Although in some patients, it is known as an initial factor, parafunctional habits can be aggravated by stress, anxiety, sleeping and eating disorder. [1,2]

2.3.2. Anatomical factors

Anatomical factors affecting the TMJ can be hereditary, developmental or acquired. Some skeletal disorders such as small mandibular arch, class II occlusion etc. can affect the TMJ. However, millimetric changes in face vertical dimension, overbite, over jet or cross bite alone, are not the only cause of TMD. Today it is believed that dental occlusion disorders are second in importance.

2.3.3. Pathophysiological factors

These include: degenerative disorders, endocrine disorders, infections and blood disorders. It is revealed that viscosity of synovial liquid and its lack of lubricant property may be the initial cause of internal derangement and clicking.

2.3.4. Mental factors

Stress and mental stresses, can result in excessive load on masticatory system and parafunctional habits. Mental and emotional disorders can be predisposing TMD causes. So, it is highly important to consider the socio-mental factors upon examination of patients with TMD.

3. Temporomandibular disorders classification

Classifying TMDs, makes diagnosis easier. As there are numerous similar disorders and pains in the head and neck region, differential diagnosis is paramount (Table 1).

1. Deviation in form
2. Disc displacement with reduction
3. Disc displacement without reduction
4. Dislocation
5. **Inflammatory conditions:**   Synovitis   Capsulitis
6. **Arthritides**:   Osteoarthrosis   Osteoarthritides   Polyarthritides
7. **Ankylosis**:   Fibrosis   Bony

Table 1. Classifying temporomandibular disorders

In differential diagnosis of TMJ disorders and pains, problems such as neoplasms, migraine, neuralgia and mental disorders should be considered. Moreover, it is noticeable that, growth-developmental disorders include aplasia, hypoplasia, hyperplasia and dysplasia can lead to TMJ problems.

Aplasia is defective growth of skull or mandible bones. These belong to one group of mandibular anomalies named hemifacial microsomia or first and second brachial arch syndrome. These are the most common developmental defects which have no articular fossa or eminence and the patient suffers from hearing problems.

Hypoplasia is low or incomplete growth of bones which is congenital or acquired. This is milder than aplasia. Many craniofacial anomalies include incomplete growth of cranial and mandibular bones, for example Treacher-Collins syndrome.

Hyperplasia is extensive growth of bones in congenital or acquired form which is unilateral in mandibular body, coronoid or condyle and leads to asymmetry. [1-3]

Dysplasia or fibrosis dysplasia is a benign disorder with defective mandible or maxilla growth which demonstrates itself as fibrotic connective growth. On radiography, it varies from lucent to ground glass.

Neoplasia may be benign or malignant. From the benign ones, osteoma, chondroma, osteoblastoma, chondroblastoma, ameloblastoma and synovial chondromatosis (which is common in TMJ) can be named. Malignant tumors such as osteosarcoma, Ewing sarcoma, chondrosarcoma, fibrosarcoma and adenocarcinoma are usually rare. About 1% of malignant tumors metastasize to jaws.

Fractures can result in displacement, damage of joint surfaces, ligaments and disc in combination with bleeding, then adhesion, or joint derangement can be expected.

In general, intrajoint disorders are divided into 6 classes:

1. Joint deformation (deviation in form)

2. Disc displacement which itself divided into: reducing and nonreducing

3. Joint dislocation

4. Inflammation

5. Articular bone inflammation (arthritides)

6. Ankylosis

Joint deformation is a mechanical painless disorder or deviation in the form of internal hard and soft tissues which may be developmental or acquired. Deviation in form is due to destructive forces resulting in physiologic deformation. Any growth or acquired remodeling and anatomic deformation that destroy joint surfaces results in mechanical interference that clinically results in joint noises or clicking during opening and closing.

Diagnostic criteria:

1. One of the most important signs of this disorder is deviation of the jaw on mouth opening and closing.

2. Complaint of mandibular movements. (i.e. locking or dislocation)

3. Repeatable joint noises during mandibular opening and closing.

4. Radiographic findings may demonstrate bony changes or deviation in joint form (i.e. flattening of condyle head or fossa)

Disc displacement: Disc displacement is the most common TMD in which the disc is displaced anteriorly. It may be with or without reduction.

Disc displacement or dislocation with reduction: Normal relationship between disc and condyle is altered on mouth opening. The disc is anterior to the condyle corrected upon translating (opening) and a click may be heard. Upon closing the condyle slips posteriorly and reaches the retrodiscal tissue and reduces. Usually, a second noise is also heard just before mouth closing but with less sound. These two noises or clicks are named reciprocal which are the results of disc displacement. As disc dislocation with reduction is common, some consider it as physiological. So, there may be no need to treat in a painless disorder. If any pain exists, it will be seen upon joint movements usually upon reduction. Severe trauma plays an important role especially in cases resulting in distraction or ruptured ligaments or capsule (Fig. 2, 3). [1,2]

Diagnostic criteria:

1. If pain exists, it becomes severe upon joint movements.

2. Repeatable noise usually upon opening and closing.

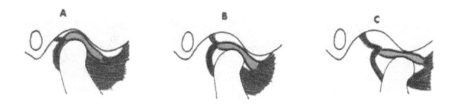

Figure 2. Normal relationship between condyle and disc; they move together.

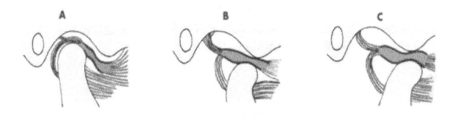

Figure 3. Disc displacement with reduction.

3.   MRI images demonstrate disc dislocation which is greater upon opening.

Disc displacement or dislocation without reduction: In this state there is alteration in translating movements and an abnormal relationship remains in opening and closing. Thus, the disc does not return to its correct position and remains dislocated anteriorly without any correction during translating movement. The term "closed lock" is used to describe this disorder (the jaw is locked and will not open). The disc is stuck anterior to the condyle and maximum opening is only 10 to 15 mm. The type of condyle and disc movement is only rotational (hinge movement). During opening, the mandible deviates to the affected side. In lateral movements, inflammation and derangement is present in posterior disc tissues. Joint noises are absent here. In acute cases, pain becomes severe by forced mandibular movements. In chronic cases, pain is distinctively less and in many patients, there is no pain. In chronic cases, a history of joint noises and then limitation in mandibular opening is usually present (Fig.4). [1,2]

Diagnostic criteria: (acute type)

1.   Pain accelerates during forced mandibular movements.

2.   Mouth opening movements are limited (hinge movement only).

3.   Deviation to the affected site exists upon mandibular opening.

4.   Limitation exists in lateral movements.

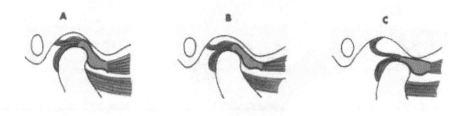

Figure 4. Anterior disc displacement without reduction-there is no translational movement.

5.   Soft tissue MRI reveals nonreducing disc displacement.

Acute disc displacement must be treated urgently by pulling the mandible downward and forward to allow the disc to "pop" in place posteriorly.

Diagnostic criteria: (chronic type)

1.   Pain if exists, is less than acute type.

2.   History of joint noises then mouth opening limitation

3.   There is mandibular opening limitation

4.   There is lateral movement limitation

5.   MRI images demonstrate nonreducing disc displacement

Mandibular dislocation is a situation in which the condyle is displaced anteriorly in front of the articular eminence and is unable to return to its normal position. To describe it, the term "open lock" is used as the mouth locks in open position (Fig. 5) .

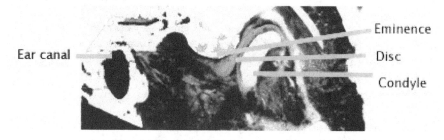

Figure 5. Mandibular dislocation - the position of the condyle head is in front of the articular eminence.

It is caused by:

1.   Disc-condyle mandibular hypermobility.

2.   Excessive translating movement of the condyle.

3. Atrophied articular eminence.

Acute mandibular dislocation must be treated urgently by pulling the mandible downward and backward to allow the condyle to "pop" in place posteriorly.

Diagnostic criteria

1. Closing Disability

2. Pain, if acute

Inflammation: Initial inflammation is rare and usually presents as rheumatologic disorders. Inflammation including synovitis, capsulitis and retrodiscitis often occur following trauma, damage, infection or other joint disorders. Pain in these disorders is acute and occurs with other joint movements.

Synovitis: Wearing of synovial tissue of TMJ can occur after trauma, intracapsular irritation and even unusual function. Clinical features of synovitis are local pain which becomes severe during mandibular movements. In many cases, fluctuant swelling in synovitis and pain inhibits posterior teeth from occluding.

Capsulitis: Capsular inflammation may occur because of distraction of capsular ligaments. Differential diagnosis of capsulitis from synovitis is difficult. It is painful. There is tenderness to palpation. The most important cause of capsulitis is macro- trauma. It is impossible to differentiate between capsulitis from synovitis clinically.

Retrodiscitis: Inflammation and degeneration is possible following excessive forces on retrodiscal tissues replete with nerves and vessels. As with other inflammations, it appears as dull pain upon clenching. Both of mild and severe traumas are causative factors. Sudden trauma to the chin results in condyle pressure on retrodiscal tissues and thus, inflammation and degeneration may occur in the long-term.

Diagnostic criteria

1. Local concentrated pain at rest which becomes severe in function and clenching

2. There is limitation in mandibular movement because of pain. Sometimes, swallowing leads to no contact of posterior teeth on that side. MRI may demonstrate inflammation.

3. If there is inflammation in the joint and teeth cannot occlude on the affected side.

Joint inflammations: They may be local, diffuse or generalized.

- Osteoarthrosis
- Osteoarthritis

Diffuse type includes: Polyarthritis which itself has 6 groups:

- Traumatic arthritis
- Infectious arthritis
- Rheumatoid arthritis

- Hyperuricemia arthritis
- Psoriatic arthritis
- Ankylosing arthritis

Osteoarthrosis: This is known as a degenerative noninflammatory condition of the joint. As we know, functional forces entering joint surfaces result in remodeling stimulation to adaptation of the condyle during life. It is a natural reaction of subjoint bone. However, if forces are more than adaptive capacity and condyle remodeling, degeneration or osteoarthritis will appear. In milder forces to joint surfaces and bone remodeling with no symptoms, it is named osteoarthrosis as conditions are stable but the shape of bone changes.

Clinical observations

It is painless. Limitation in mandibular movements and deviation to the affected side occurs on opening.

Radiographic findings

Bone remodeling, changes in shape and size which are signs of physiologic adaptive mechanical stress are seen. However, initial degeneration of joint can be demonstrated with arthroscopy.

Diagnostic criteria

1. Crepitus, (grating sound)
2. Limitation in mandibular movements resulting in deviation to the affected side on opening.
3. If radiography shows bony changes, they include: subchondral sclerosis, osteophyte, density loss, subjoint cysts.

Osteoarthritis: This is a degenerative condition sometimes associated with a secondary inflammation of the TMJ (i.e. synovitis). Osteoarthritis is a degenerative process of condyle and fossa surfaces resulting in their changes. It has slow progression then cartilage remodels and reshapes. Osteoarthritis may be a component of a systemic disorder.

Etiology

When articular surfaces are unable to bear the forces, the capacity of functional adaptation cannot respond and thus, degeneration ensues. If bony changes are active, it is named osteoarthritis.

Clinical features

Limitation of opening is present because of articular pain. Crepitus is obviously common. Condyle palpation leads to pain.

Radiographic findings

Include: bony changes in subarticular bone of condyle and fossa, sclerosis, subarticular cysts, osteophyte, low density and roughness. In progressive conditions, extensive condyle degeneration is present. It is considerable that patient may have signs before demineralization in radiography. Individuals suffering from osteoarthritis usually have unilateral pain which becomes worsened in mandibular movements and also in late afternoon and night. Articular changes may be due to trauma, destructive forces, infection or an idiopathic process (Fig. 6).

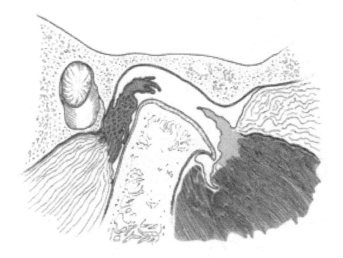

Figure 6. Degenerative lesions in the TMJ with disc perforation.

Diagnostic criteria:

1. Pain upon function due to inflammation.

2. Trigger points to palpation are present.

3. Crepitus

4. Limitation in mandibular movements with deviation to the affected side on opening

5. Radiographic changes include : subchondral sclerosis, osteophyte, narrowing of articular space

Polyarthritides: This includes a variety of articular disorders which are less common. Their signs and symptoms are like in osteoarthritis but with completely different etiology. Different types include: Traumatic arthritis, infectious arthritis, rheumatoid arthritis, hyperuricemia arthritis, psoriatic arthritis and ankylosing arthritis.

Traumatic arthritis: Major trauma to the jaw leads to articular surface changes and inflammation. Clinically, patients have consistent pain becoming severe with movements and opening limitation.

Infection Arthritis: It occurs because of bacterial infection from adjacent structures.

Rheumatoid arthritis: It is an autoimmune chronic systemic disorder which leads to synovitis. Clinical features are continuous pain, pain on swallowing and limitation in mandibular movements. It involves joints of the legs, at first. In 5%, there are signs in the TMJ. In about 80% of patients, rheumatoid factor is positive. In initial stages, there is no distinctive radiographic sign because changes are in soft tissues. But after progressing, erosive changes, subchondral cysts, decrease in articular space, bone degeneration and osteoporosis can be seen. In acute cases, inflammation and tenderness to palpation is present. Limitation in mandibular movement leads to ankylosis progress. Condyle degeneration may result in VD reduction and anterior open bite. Crepitus or joint noises may be present, also. Histologically, in progressive stages, there is severe secretion of lymphocytes, plasma cells and lysosomic enzymes with exudates in the joint. It usually affects the TMJs bilaterally and is more common in women (Fig. 7).

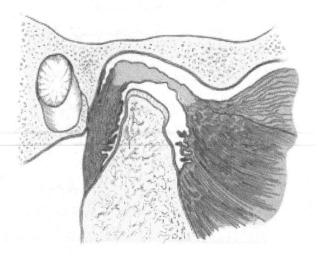

Figure 7. Degenerative changes in rheumatoid arthritis-attenuation of the condyle.

Hyperuricemia: In this disorder, crystals of sodium urate in periarticular tissues increase which lead to, warmness, tenderness to palpation and pain in mandibular movement. Gout is a common hereditary disease in men. In laboratory tests, uric acid and erythrocyte sedimentation rate in blood is high. In radiography, punch-out bone erosions can be seen.

Psoriatic arthritis: This is an autoimmune disease accompanied by psoriasis dermatic lesions. Psoriatic arthritis affects men more than women and Rh factor is negative. Radiographic findings reveal osteoarthritis changes with erosion, osteoporosis and narrowing of articular space. This polyarthritis is asymmetric. Joint signs are pain, warmness, pain on swallowing and limitation in mandibular movements.

Ankylosing spondylitis: Ankylosing spondylitis or Marie-Strumpel disease is a chronic inflammatory disease with unknown cause.There is HLA-B27 marker. It involves joints of the vertebrae. There is calcification in ligaments tending toward bony ankylosis here. It is more common in men. There are signs such as arthritis and iridocyclitis present. The possibility of involving TMJ is low but in cases of TMJ involvement, signs are mild and the most important one of them is limitation in mandibular movements, pain, and diffuse stiffness in muscles. These patients have severe signs in other joints. On radiography, bone margins of subchondral bone are absent and sclerosis, bony erosions, narrowing of joint space and extensive ankylosis are visible.

Ankylosis: In general, ankylosis means abnormal immobility of the jaw and mandibular movements because of adhesion. It is divided into 2 major groups: bony and fibrotic. In fibrotic ankylosis fibrous adhesion or fibrotic changes in capsular ligaments occurs. It is the most common form which occurs between condyle and disc or between disc and fossa. Bony ankylosis occurs between condyle and glenoid fossa, and leads to fusion. In another classification, low mobility disorders are divided into three groups:

Trismus because of stiffness of masticatory muscles.

1. Psudoankylosis which results from extracapsular causes and leads to reduced mandibular movements.

2. True ankylosis: It results from fibrosis adhesion or bony fusion. The most severe form of it is low mobility because of bony adhesion of condyle to glenoid fossa.

The most common form of low mobility is trismus from infection, trauma, malocclusion, tumors and mental problems.

The most common cause of pseudoankylosis is due to zygomatic arch and condyle fracture. This fracture leads to transgression of a part of these structures to articular space and finally, inhibition of condyle movements. Adhesion of the coronoid process and hypertrophy around it, or fibrosis of the temporalis muscle, can be considered as other causes of pseudo ankylosis. In true ankylosis, trauma is the most common cause of bony ankylosis. Following trauma, in children, after 3 to 6 months, mandibular movements become progressively reduced; the most important mechanism after trauma, is bone formation following intracapsular hematoma or intracapsular fracture. The most important cause of ankylosis after trauma is intracapsular infection. With a lower percentage, ankylosis occurs after intracapsular inflammations such as rheumatoid arthritis, Still's disease, Marie-Strumpel disease etc. Fibrosis or bony ankylosis is also common after arthroplasty. Bony type occurs after diskectomy as well. In initial diagnosis, panoramic radiography can be used. More complete information is gained from CT scans. If fibrotic ankylosis is present, articular space decreases. Articular space loss is a sign of disc destruction; the space may fill with bone. [1,4]

Etiology: The most common cause of is macrotrauma which leads to tissue damage, inflammation and hemarthrosis. These increase the formation of fibrous matrix. The other cause of ankylosis is surgery that often results in fibrotic changes and reduced mandibular movements. Fibrosis ankylosis of mandible is the continuous progression of joint adhesion.

Clinical features: Patients have history of damage or capsulitis with reduced mandibular movements (which is painless). Mandibular movements in all directions (opening, lateral and protrusive) are limited. If ankylosis is unilateral, the jaw deviates to the affected site on opening. In most cases of ankylosis, the condyle can rotate to some degree thus the patient is able to open his/her mouth 20 to 25 mm. Bilateral ankylosis in children results in severe retrognathia and bird face with open bite.

Diagnostic criteria (fibrosis type):

1. Reduced opening limit

2. Distinctive deviation to the affected site

3. There is no translational movement of condyle

Diagnostic criteria (bony type):

1. Severe mandibular movements limitation

2. Deviation to the affected site in unilateral cases

3. When it is unilateral, lateral movements to the unaffected site is clearly limited.

4. Bony proliferation and immobility of the condyle on radiography (Fig. 8).

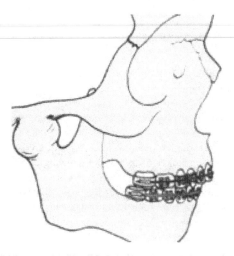

Figure 8. Complete bony ankylosis

Adhesion: Sticking of joint surfaces to each other may occur between condyle and disc (inferior articular space) or between disc and glenoid fossa (superior articular space). This may follow long-term forces (for example clenching during sleep), hemarthrosis, macro trauma and or surgery.

Clinical features:

In adhesion between disc and fossa, normal translational movement is limited, so the condyle just has rotational movement. In this case, opening range is about 25 to 30 mm.

If this kind of adhesion occurs permanently in the superior joint space, the disc remains posterior to the condyle which in fact is posterior dislocation of the disc.

In adhesions of the inferior joint space, translational movements may be normal. But the condyle is unable to do rotational movement with the disc. The result is a jolt during mouth opening.

Masticatory muscles disorders

Masticatory muscles disorders in the head and neck region, include: myofacial pains, myositis, spasm, protective splinting, contracture and neoplasia. In most patients with TMD, the muscles are tender to palpation and 40% of them have pain chewing food. Fibromyalgia is a chronic muscle pain.

Myofacial pain

Myofacial pain can be misleading by tension type headache resulting from tiredness.

Etiology :

The most important causes are : Systemic factors such as vitamin deficiency, viral infection, mental stress and sleep disorders. The chief compliant of the patient is various pains, recurrent pains, temporal headache etc. Here, the patients show the site of pain not the source of it.

Clinical features:

The most important sign of myofacial pains is trigger point.Other signs are pain at rest and upon activity.

Diagnostic criteria:

1. Poorly localized pain

2. Localized trigger point in muscles or fascia

3. Pain decrease in localized anesthetic injection

Myositis or inflammatory myalgia

This is a muscular tissue inflammation resulting from localized causes such as trauma or infection. Myositis is divided in two types of inflammatory reactions:.

Diagnostic criteria: (type 1)

1. Pain increase in mandibular movements

2. Pain following long and abnormal use of muscles

Diagnostic criteria: (type 2 : diffuse)

1. Pain is usually acute in localized areas

2. Localized tenderness to palpation in all parts of the muscles

3. Pain increase in mandibular movements

4. Moderate to severe limited movements due to inflammation

Myospasm or tonic contraction myalgia:

Myospasm is a toxic muscular contraction created by CNS

Myospasm or acute trismus is an acute disorder and sudden and involuntary contraction.

Diagnostic criteria:

1. Acute pain

2. Persistent contraction of muscle

3. Hyperactivity of EMG

4. Pain decrease in activity

5. Pain at rest and tenderness to palpation

Evaluation and diagnosis of temporomandibular disorders

The patient history should include chief complaint, history of the present illness, medical and dental history and individual history (Table 2).

1. Do you have difficulty, pain or both when opening your mouth, for instance when yawing?
2. Does your jaw stick, locked, or go out?
3. Do you have difficulty, pain or both when chewing, talking or using your jaws?
4. Are you aware of noises on the jaw joint?
5. Do your jaws regularly feel stiff, tight or tired?
6. Do you have pain in or about the ears, temples or cheeks?
7. Do you have frequent headaches and or neck aches?
8. Have you had a recent injury to your head, neck or jaw?
9. Have you been aware of any recent changes in your bite?
10. Have you previously been treated for a jaw joint problem? If so when?
Masticatory muscle disorders
1. Myofacial pain
2. Myositis
3. Spasm

4. Protective splinting

5. Contracture

6. Neoplasia

Usual examinations in TMD

1. Measure range of motion of the mandible or opening and right and left lateral excursions (note any uncoordination in the movement)

2. Palpate for pre- auricular or interameatal TMJ tenderness

3. Auscultate and or palpate for TMJ sounds (clicking or crepitus)

4. Palpate for tenderness in the masseter and temporalis muscle

5. Note excessive occlusal wear , excessive tooth mobility , buccal mucosal lateral tongue scalloping

6. Inspect symmetry and arrangement of the face, jaw and dental arches

Differential diagnosis of oral and maxillofacial pains:

1. Intracranial structures

2. Extracranial structures

3. Neuromuscular disorders

4. Neuropathic pain disorders

5. Continuous pain disorders

6. Sympathetic maintained pain

7. Psychogenic pain disorders

8. Somatoform disorders

Pseudoankylosis :

1. Depressed zygomatic arch fracture

2. Fracture dislocation of the condyle

3. Adhesions of the coronoid process

4. Hyper trophy of the coronoid process

5. Fibrosis of the temporalis muscle

6. Myositis ossificans

7. Scar contracture following thermal injury

8. Tumor of the condyle or coronoid process

True ankylosis:

1. Inter capsular fracture (child)

2. Medial displaced condylar fracture (adult)

3. Obstetric trauma

4. Intracapsular fibrosis

5. Infection : otitis media		
6. Suppurative arthritis		
7. Inflammation:,	Rheumatoid arthritis	Stills disease
8. Ankylosing spondylitis		
9. Mari Strumpel disease		
Surgical : Post operative complications of TMJ surgery Orthognathic surgery		

Hypomobility of the mandible

1. Odontogenic :myofacial pain , malocclusion , erupting teeth
2. Infection: pterygomandibular , lateropharyngeal , temporal
3. Trauma: fracture of the mandible , muscle contusion
4. Tumors: nasopharyngeal tumors, tumors that invade jaw muscle
5. Psychological: hysterical trismus
6. Pharmacologic: phenothiazines
7. Neurologic: tetanus

Sign and symptoms of mental disorders

1. Inconsistent , inappropriate and or vague of pain
2. Over-dramatization of symptoms
3. Symptoms that vary with life events
4. Significant pain of greater than 6 month duration
5. Repeated failures with conventional therapies
6. Inconsistent response to medications
7. History of other stress – related disorders
8. Major life events e.g. new job , marriage , divorce , death
9. Evidence of drug abuse
10. Clinically significant anxiety or depression
11. Evidence of secondary gain

Table 2. Questionnaire about TMD

Recommended Imaging for TMD:

Panoramic view:

It is a valuable method in diagnosis of TMD. Advantages are low price and the possibility of comparing both sides of mandible and fossae.

Generally, information from panoramic view include: whole evaluation of maxilla and mandible bilaterally (coronoid process and condyle).

Magnetic Resonance Imaging (MRI):

Today, MRI often is used to diagnose of TMD. This method evaluates both joints at the same time. Video film is achieved from mandibular movements during imaging, also. On the other hand, the danger of high radiation is obviated.

Computed tomography (CT Scan):

This technique is used in recognizing bony abnormal cases or anomalies of TMJ (such as developmental anomalies, trauma and neoplasia). CT does not play an important role in diagnosing disc displacement because it is problematic in showing the disc. CT scan with direct sagittal plane provides high quality images. It is the best method in evaluating bone structures (ankylosis) in combination with TMJ.

Disadvantages:

1. High price

2. No suitable images of soft tissue within the joint

3. No possibility of imaging during motion of disc and condyle

Arthrography:

It refers to the injection of a radiopaque contrast medium into the inferior, superior or both spaces and evaluating intracapsular soft tissues. Dynamic and functional movement of the disc and condyle can be assessed via fluoroscopy and video in this method. This technique is very precise in observing intracapsular derangement. Arthrography is the method choice to recognize disc perforations.

Disadvantages:

It is a minimally invasive method, may result in infection, hematoma, disc injury, or hyper-sensitivity to the medium.

Diagnoses achieved by arthrography:

1. Disc dislocation with reduction

2. Disc dislocation without reduction

3. Perforation

4. Adhesion

Mental and socio-behavioral evaluation:

In patients with TMD especially who suffer from chronic pain sometimes stress due to muscle hyperactivity may be recognized as a major factor. So there should be some questions in order to evaluate behavioral, social and emotional factors because they may result in initiation, or exacerbation of the disorder. On the other hand, long-term chronic pains with function disorder can lead to mental changes. Anxiety and depression are recognized by simple questions.

Additional clinical tests:

Biopsy:

This is helpful in diagnosis of benign and malignant tumors of the TMJ; the most important of them are chondroma, chondrosarcoma and osteochondromatosis.

Diagnostic anesthesia injection:

These injections include:

1. Nerve block (auriculotemporal nerve)

2. Trigger points injection

3. TMJ injections

4. Conservative therapy

Treatment goals in patients with TMD are : Pain relief and return of function. These goals will be achieved only if diagnosed properly and the treatment plan takes mental and physical problems into consideration. Predisposing factors must be eliminated. In many cases, signs and symptoms of TMD are transient and self-limited without any serious sequelae and no invasive treatment is needed. [1,2]

Conservative treatments such as behavioral modifications, physiotherapy, medication therapy and splint therapy decreases signs and symptoms in most patients suffering from TMD. There are many studies that emphasize this point; 86% or more of these patients with disc displacement become pain-free and regain acceptable function. [1,2]

In general, TMD treatments are divided into two separate phases :

Phase 1: Includes education, anxiety control, behavioral modifications, medication therapy and splint therapy.

Phase 2: Dental rehabilitation, occlusion correction, fixed prosthesis, restorative treatments, orthodontic treatments and orthognathic surgery. The concept of treatment phase 2 is that it will be done automatically after completion of phase 1. In spite of successful conservative treatment in TMD, some patients do not improve. These patients are divided in two groups:

1. Pain and dysfunction is as a result of changes in joint structures. Joint surgery may be needed in this case.

2. 2- Patients with chronic syndromes or combination of factors. In this case, a treatment plan for chronic pain and a group of specialists may be needed. Selective treatments include:

3. Patient education and stress control

4. Mental therapy

5. Pharmacotherapy

6. Physiotherapy

7. Splint therapy

8. Occlusal correction

9. Surgery

Patient education and stress control: Successful treatment lies in awareness, patient motivation and cooperation. Dentist should explain clinical findings, diagnostic information, treatment choices and prognosis in simple terms. Necessary instructions should include;

1. Muscle relaxant by voluntary limitation in mandibular function

2. Parafunctional habits modification

3. Physiotherapy at home

The program should emphasize avoiding chewing hard food or gum, yawning, singing, excessive talking, bruxism and clenching and bad sleeping habits. Home physiotherapy plan includes moist warm towels on sensitive areas can decrease sensitivity and pain and also increase the range of mandibular movements. Heat relaxes muscles in the form of warm and moist compress. Patient's stress and habits can be treated by a combination of different methods such as behavioral modifications, medication therapy and physiotherapy. Patient cooperation and motivation play an important role here.

Pharmacotherapy:

It is effective in treatment of TMD. Clinical experiences show that pharmacotherapy and supportive treatment will accelerate patient improvement. It is noticeable that no drug has a complete range of effectiveness in TMD. The most effective drugs to treat all kinds of TMD include analgesics and nonsteroidal anti-inflammatory drugs (NSAIDs), corticosteroids, muscle relaxants, anti-depressants and antianxiety drugs. Analgesics and corticosteroids in acute TMD pain, nonsteroidal anti-inflammatory drugs and muscle relaxants in both acute and chronic disorders and tricyclic anti- depressants in chronic problems are recommended. It is advised that tranquillizing drugs three times a day for two weeks be given.

Analgesic drugs:

These drugs are used to decrease pain in TMD. Non-narcotics are effective on mild to moderate pains. The primary form aspirin inhibits prostaglandin synthesis. Ibuprofen is effective in skeletomuscular pains (dosage: 600 – 800 mg three times daily). These drugs may have gastrointestinal side-effects.

Corticosteroids:

These drugs have effective anti-inflammatory properties but rarely used in TMD.

Muscle relaxant drugs:

These drugs are advised for muscle hyperactivity inhibition in TMD; mainly benzodiazapines.

Anti depressant drugs:

Recently, antidepressant drugs are used in different kinds of chronic pains. For example, pain decrease is expected in low dose of Amitriptyline (Elavil) 10 mg before sleep for some weeks. This 1/10 to 1/20 dosage is because of its antidepressant property.This drug can be used in individuals who have depression and sleep disorder due to their chronic pain and is effective in treatment of headache resulting from muscle contraction and musculoskeletal pains. It increases the stage 4 (delta) of sleep and reduces rapid eye movement (REM) in sleep. They may be effective in treatment of nightly bruxism, also. In dosage between 10 to 75 mg, they are effective in treatment of orofacial chronic pains. Antidepressant drugs should be advised by specialists. Recommendations of these drugs are for individuals who have depression not only TMD.

Antianxiety drugs:

They are effective when TMD is associated with anxiety. They reduce the patient's reaction to stress. The most common drugs in this group is diazepam which should not be given for more than 10 days. Dosage of 2.5 to 5 mg before sleeping results in muscle relaxation and probable decrease in parafunctional habits.

Local anesthetic drugs:

As it was said before, local anesthetic drugs are used for two aims of treating and diagnosing. When we are suspecting neuralgia, or treating disc or mandibular dislocations. [5,6]

Physical therapy:

A group of supportive treatments used as an important part of successful treatment of TMD includes physiotherapy.

Physical therapy modalities: This treatment includes: Thermal therapy, ultrasound, electro-galvanic stimulation therapy, low voltage electric stimulation, acupuncture and low-level laser. [7]

Thermal therapy:

Heat leads to blood flow increase at that site. A moist warm towel can be used in the site for 10-15 minutes, on and off.

Ultra sound:

This method results in increasing temperature of internal tissue surfaces, so deep surfaces become warmer. Its mechanism is translating high frequency to heat during passing through tissues. This heat is able to penetrate.

Splint therapy: 1 – Interocclusal splint, 2 – Anterior repositioning splint

Splints solves muscle tension and TMJ pain decreases. In anterior displacement of disc and degenerative joint disorder, splint decreases direct pressure in TMJ area so joint and muscles have a passive state. Occlusal splints use in TMD treatments as temporary and conservative treatment decrease occlusal direct load in TMJ region. It allows the patient to seek the most comfortable muscle and joint position without excessive influence of the occlusion. It is advised to use the splint at night for several months because results appear then. Theoretically, the position of disc and condyle head is corrected and condyle is placed in a proper relation with the disc. So, posterior disc ligaments shorten maintaining the disc in proper relationship to the condyle. However, splints may be required for a year or more to stabilize treatment, provide relief pain and discomfort of TMJ (Figs. 9, 10).

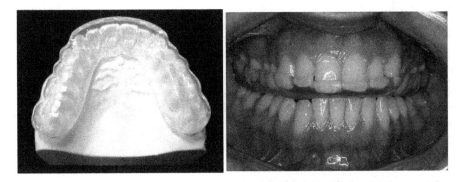

Figure 9. Maxillary hard acrylic splint.

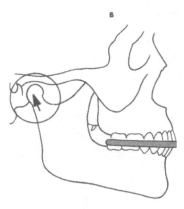

Figure 10. Maxillary hard acrylic splint increases joint space when used; it allows for disc reduction, relieves spasms, redistributes occlusal forces and prevents attrition.

5. TMJ surgery

Although most patients with TMJ disorders can be treated by nonsurgical and conservative treatment, in some, surgery is necessary. The common TMJ surgeries are:

1. Arthrocentesis

2. Arthroscopy

3. Disc – repositioning surgery

4. Condylotomy

5. Arthroplasty

6. Total joint displacement

Arthrocentesis:

Arthrocentesis involves placing a suitable needle into the superior joint space and aspiration for histopathology examinations, and then a large amount of lactated Ringer's solution is injected into the superior joint space to debride the superior joint space. This is done by a maxillofacial surgeon who has enough skill and experience in TMJ surgery to prevent adverse effects. Most patients undergoing arthrocentesis prefer local anesthesia and sedation.

Arthroscopy

Use of arthroscopy in diagnosing, treating and surgery of TMJ disorders is very popular. In comparison with open surgery and direct cutting of local tissues, arthroscopy is more comfortable with less adverse effects. In Arthroscopy, at first, a small cannula is placed into the superior joint space, followed by insertion of an arthroscope with a light source.The end of arthroscope is connected to a TV and a video monitor which allows perfect visualization of all aspects of the joint including glenoid fossa and joint disc. Intrajoint space just can be visualized and joint space can be washed and pathologic adhesions can be lysed. One cannula is used for visualization, where as instruments are placed through the other one are instruments such as forceps, scissors, sutures, cautery, medication needles, laser instrumentation and shavers. So, Arthroscopy is possible for disc displacement, disc attachment release, posterior band cautery, and suture techniques.Laser fibers can also be used to eliminate adhesions and inflamed tissue and cutting adhesions. A variety of TMJ disorders, including internal disorders, hypomobility as a result of fibrotic adhesions, DJD, hypermobility or excessive movements of joint can be treated by arthroscopy.

It is noteworthy that before and after arthroscopy, conservative treatments such as splint therapy and physiotherapy are used (Fig. 11).

Disc repair:

In advanced disorders, the joint disc may be severely damaged. Sometimes it can be repaired but in other cases there is no alternative except to remove it. Disc repair or replacement is done with autogenous grafts include dermis, temporalis fascia, auricular cartilage or inferior nasal

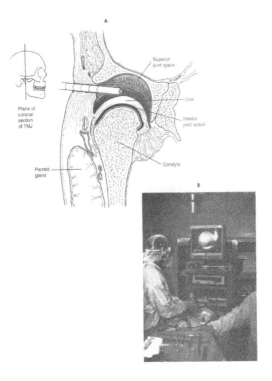

Figure 11. Arthroscopy of the superior joint space.

concha. Although, long-term results of these methods are not desirable in all cases, but most patients are satisfied from local function improvement and pain decrease.

Condylotomy of TMJ:

In this method, a subcondylar osteotomy in the ramus is used which starts from the sigmoid notch and ends inferiorly to the condylar neck. The lateral pterygoid muscle pulls the head of the condyle in a new passive relationship with disc and joint socket. It is suggested in some disorders such as recurrent anterior disc displacement and in degenerative joint disease.

Arthroplasty:

It is a treatment choice in bony ankylosis and fibrosis of TMJ. In this method, a part of the condyle head is removed. A gap is created between the head of the condyle and glenoid fossa so the patient can open his/her mouth.[4]

Total joint replacement:

Sometimes, advanced degenerative lesions lead to condyle process destruction, so it is necessary to repair that part by autogenous graft or other implants. In advanced rheumatoid arthritis, neoplastic lesions, trauma and damage to local structures, there are destructions in many parts of the condyle and glenoid fossa. Costochondral graft often is used to replace condyle head and neck. In total joint replacement, titanium is used which has the same shape as the glenoid fossa and condyle head. This avoids severe pains, limitation or ankylosis, complete closed lock, deformation and severe malocclusion. (Fig.12)

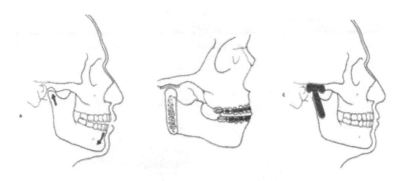

Figure 12. Total joint replacement – condyle removal and replacement via prosthesis.

Myofacial pain dysfunction syndrome (MPDS)

Causes pain, discomfort and inflammation in muscles and joints affecting function and activity of the masticatory system. This is a maxillofacial muscle disorder due to parafunctional habits or muscular hyperactivity and because of stress and anxiety.

Methods of stress control include: Exercise, avoiding stressful factors, psychological consultant, behavioral modification, soft diet for 4 weeks, trying to maximum opening the mouth without pressure, pain, slowly and with stretching exercises.

Medication:

1.   Analgesic and anti inflammatory drugs

Ibuprofen – piroxicam, or acetaminophen codeine 3 – 4 times daily for 10 – 14 days

2.   Muscle relaxant :

In individuals with muscles hyperactivity and severe pain give (3 -4 times daily for 10 – 14 days) diazepam (2- 5 mg 3 – 4 times in a day).

2.   Tricyclic anti – depressant such as Amitriptyline (Elavil) lead to sleep improvement, nightly bruxism decreases and muscle pain improvement.

Triptizol Tab 10 – 25 mg, nightly before sleep

Physical therapy: Includes: Relaxation therapy, Ultrasound heating, stretching, pressure massage

Permanent occlusion modification:

After a reversible and conservative treatment, some people need permanent treatment and occlusal adjustment. It includes: prosthetic restoration, orthodontic treatment, orthognathic surgery and occlusal equilibration if it is necessary. These treatments in indicated patients may provide long-term treatment effects.

Surgical treatments include:

Arthrocentesis, Arthroscopy, Disc repair or removal, Disc repositioning, Condylotomy, Total joint replacement.

Author details

Fina Navi[1], Mohammad Hosein Kalantar Motamedi[3], Koroush Taheri Talesh[2], Esshagh Lasemi[2] and Zahra Nematollahi[4]

1 Scientific Faculty, Department of Oral and Maxillofacial Surgery, Azad University of Medical Sciences, Tehran, Iran

2 Department of Oral and Maxillofacial Surgery, Azad University of Medical Sciences, Tehran, Iran

3 Department of Oral and Maxillofacial Surgery, Trauma Research Center, Baqiyatallah University of Medical Sciences, Tehran, Iran

4 Private Practice Dentistry, Tehran, Iran

References

[1] Dowlat Abadi MMotamedi MHK, Taheri KT. Textbook of Temporomandibular Disorders. Shayan Nemodar Publications, Tehran, (2009). , 2009, 5-100.

[2] Mortazavi, S. H. Motamedi MHK, Navi F, Pourshahab M, Bayanzadeh SM, Hajmiragha H, Isapour M: Outcomes of management of early temporomandibular joint disorders: How effective is nonsurgical therapy in the long-term? National J Maxillofac Surg, (2010).

[3] Motamedi, M. H. Treatment of condylar hyperplasia of the mandible using unilateral ramus osteotomies. J Oral Maxillofac Surg. (1996). Oct;discussion 1169-70, 54(10), 1161-9.

[4] Behnia, H, Motamedi, M. H, & Tehranchi, A. Use of activator appliances in pediatric patients treated with costochondral grafts for temporomandibular joint ankylosis: analysis of 13 cases. J Oral Maxillofac Surg. (1997). discussion 1414-6., 55, 1408-14.

[5] Motamedi, M. H, Rahmat, H, Bahrami, E, Sadidi, A, Navi, F, Asadollahi, M, & Eshke-vari, P. S. Trigeminal neuralgia and radiofrequency. Todays FDA. (2010). Sep-Oct; 22(5):54-5, 57-9.

[6] Bohluli, B, Motamedi, M. H, Bagheri, S. C, Bayat, M, Lassemi, E, Navi, F, & Mohar-amnejad, N. Use of botulinum toxin A for drug-refractory trigeminal neuralgia: pre-liminary report.Oral Surg Oral Med Oral Pathol Oral Radiol Endod. (2011). Jan;Epub 2010 Jul 31, 111(1), 47-50.

[7] Lassemi, E, & Jafari, S. M. Motamedi MHK, Navi F, Lasemi R: Low-level Laser Thera-pie in the Management of Temporomandibular Joint Disorder. JOLA, (2008).

Permissions

The contributors of this book come from diverse backgrounds, making this book a truly international effort. This book will bring forth new frontiers with its revolutionizing research information and detailed analysis of the nascent developments around the world.

We would like to thank Mohammad Hosein Kalantar Motamedi, DDS, for lending his expertise to make the book truly unique. He has played a crucial role in the development of this book. Without his invaluable contribution this book wouldn't have been possible. He has made vital efforts to compile up to date information on the varied aspects of this subject to make this book a valuable addition to the collection of many professionals and students.

This book was conceptualized with the vision of imparting up-to-date information and advanced data in this field. To ensure the same, a matchless editorial board was set up. Every individual on the board went through rigorous rounds of assessment to prove their worth. After which they invested a large part of their time researching and compiling the most relevant data for our readers. Conferences and sessions were held from time to time between the editorial board and the contributing authors to present the data in the most comprehensible form. The editorial team has worked tirelessly to provide valuable and valid information to help people across the globe.

Every chapter published in this book has been scrutinized by our experts. Their significance has been extensively debated. The topics covered herein carry significant findings which will fuel the growth of the discipline. They may even be implemented as practical applications or may be referred to as a beginning point for another development. Chapters in this book were first published by InTech; hereby published with permission under the Creative Commons Attribution License or equivalent.

The editorial board has been involved in producing this book since its inception. They have spent rigorous hours researching and exploring the diverse topics which have resulted in the successful publishing of this book. They have passed on their knowledge of decades through this book. To expedite this challenging task, the publisher supported the team at every step. A small team of assistant editors was also appointed to further simplify the editing procedure and attain best results for the readers.

Our editorial team has been hand-picked from every corner of the world. Their multi-ethnicity adds dynamic inputs to the discussions which result in innovative outcomes. These outcomes are then further discussed with the researchers and contributors who give their valuable feedback and opinion regarding the same. The feedback is then collaborated with the researches and they are edited in a comprehensive manner to aid the understanding of the subject.

Apart from the editorial board, the designing team has also invested a significant amount of their time in understanding the subject and creating the most relevant covers. They scrutinized every image to scout for the most suitable representation of the subject and create an appropriate cover for the book.

The publishing team has been involved in this book since its early stages. They were actively engaged in every process, be it collecting the data, connecting with the contributors or procuring relevant information. The team has been an ardent support to the editorial, designing and production team. Their endless efforts to recruit the best for this project, has resulted in the accomplishment of this book. They are a veteran in the field of academics and their pool of knowledge is as vast as their experience in printing. Their expertise and guidance has proved useful at every step. Their uncompromising quality standards have made this book an exceptional effort. Their encouragement from time to time has been an inspiration for everyone.

The publisher and the editorial board hope that this book will prove to be a valuable piece of knowledge for researchers, students, practitioners and scholars across the globe.

List of Contributors

Jeong Keun Lee
Department of Dentistry Oral and Maxillofacial Surgery, Ajou University School of Medicine, Suwon, Korea

Yong Seok Cho
Apseon Dental Hospital, Seoul, Korea

Hany A. Emam
Oral and Maxillofacial Surgery Department, Georgia Health Sciences University, Augusta, Georgia, USA
Oral and Maxillofacial Surgery, Cairo University, Egypt

Mark R. Stevens
Oral and Maxillofacial Surgery Department, Georgia Health Sciences University, Augusta, Georgia, USA

Ali Hassani
Oral and Maxillofacial Surgery, Azad University of Medical Sciences, Tehran, Iran

Mohammad Hosein Kalantar Motamedi
Oral and Maxillofacial Surgery, Trauma Research Center, Baqiyatallah University of Medical Sciences, Tehran, Iran

Sarang Saadat
Craniomaxillofacial Research Center, Tehran University of Medical Sciences, Tehran, Iran

Kazuma Fujimura and Kazuhisa Bessho
Department of Oral and Maxillofacial Surgery, Graduate School of Medicine, Kyoto University, Kyoto, Japan

F. Arcuri, M. Giarda, L. Stellin, A. Gatti, M. Nicolotti, M. Brucoli and A. Benech
Department of Maxillo-Facial Surgery, Novara Major Hospital: University of Eastern Piedmont "Amedeo Avogadro", Novara, Italy

P. Boffano
University of Turin, Italy

Jan Rustemeyer
Department of Oral and Maxillofacial Surgery, Klinikum Bremen-Mitte, School of Medicine of the University of Göttingen, Germany

Mehmet Cemal Akay
Ege University, Faculty of Dentistry, Department of Oral and Maxillofacial Surgery, Izmir, Turkey

Fina Navi
Scientific Faculty, Department of Oral and Maxillofacial Surgery, Azad University of Medical Sciences, Tehran, Iran

Esshagh Lasemi and Koroush Taheri Talesh
Department of Oral and Maxillofacial Surgery, Azad University of Medical Sciences, Tehran, Iran

Zahra Nematollahi
Private Practice Dentistry, Tehran, Iran

Printed in the USA
CPSIA information can be obtained
at www.ICGtesting.com
JSHW011350221024
72173JS00003B/249